Alzheimer's Disease:
Caregivers Speak Out

Alzheimer's Disease: Caregivers Speak Out

A guide to understanding, caring and coping

Pam Haisman, R.N., M.S.

Nurse Consultant for Alzheimer's Disease
Fort Myers, Florida

Chippendale House Publishers
P.O. Box 07155
Fort Myers, FL 33919

ALZHEIMER'S DISEASE: CAREGIVERS SPEAK OUT

Chippendale House Publishers
P.O. Box 07155
Fort Myers, FL 33919

ISBN: 0-9662272-0-4

Printed in the United States of America
First Printing: April, 1998
Second Printing: September, 1998
Third Printing: October, 2000

Editing Assistance: Judy Krause and Liz Scott
Support Details: The National Nurses in Business Association
Preparation Design: Kevin Owen
Internet Support: Paul Haisman

Cover: On the front cover is displayed the teal-colored ribbon acknowledging Alzheimer's awareness and the hope of a cure for Alzheimer's disease and related dementias. This national campaign was organized by The Alzheimer's and Dementia CareGivers Support Group made up of husbands, wives, sons, daughters, grandchildren, brothers and sisters of victims of Alzheimer's and related dementias.

For all who are touched by Alzheimer's disease

Acknowledgments

My family encouraged me.
My colleagues empowered me.
My friends motivated me.
My husband supported me.
I am grateful for their love.

However, it is caregivers
who had the courage to speak out,
the determination to make a difference,
and the dedication to help those with Alzheimer's
who inspired me the most to complete this "labor of love"
and to whom I owe a depth of gratitude ❤

Alzheimer's Disease: Caregivers Speak Out

TABLE OF CONTENTS

Alzheimer's Disease: Caregivers Speak Out

TABLE OF CONTENTS

Alzheimer's Disease: Caregivers Speak Out

TABLE OF CONTENTS

Alzheimer's Disease: Caregivers Speak Out

TABLE OF CONTENTS

Alzheimer's Disease: Caregivers Speak Out

TABLE OF CONTENTS

Beatitudes For The Aged
By Ester Mary Walker

Blessed are they who understand
My faltering step and palsied hand.

Blessed are they who know today
My ears must strain to catch what they say.

Blessed are they who seem to know
My eyes are dim and my wits are slow.

Blessed are they that looked away
When coffee spilled at the table today.

Blessed are they with a cheery smile
Who stop to chat for a little while.
Blessed are they who never say,
"You've told me that story twice today."

Blessed are they who know the ways
To bring back memories of yesterdays.

Blessed are they who make it known
That I'm loved, respected, and not alone.

Blessed are they who know I'm at a loss
To find the strength to carry the cross.

Blessed are they who ease the days
On my journey Home in loving ways."

(Shared with permission)

INTRODUCTION

"I wish everyone understood Alzheimer's disease is the most insidious, inconceivably destructive disease to both patient and caregivers," laments one despairing family caregiver. *"Its invisibility is not at all understood like illnesses that leave scars or can be seen in a microscope. I just wish people could understand what years of gradual grieving do to a person who is losing the only other person in the world who has given unconditional love. The stress of caring for this person has meant slipping in and out of depression. How do I explain that to all of you? How can I get you to understand how I feel? I can't. So I carry on almost silently with a periodic urge to climb a hill and shout to everyone about how I feel. But I can't. You wouldn't understand anyway. How could you, when I don't understand it myself? I just wish everyone would understand . . . about Alzheimer's disease!"*

As a nurse, educator, support group facilitator, and Alzheimer's disease researcher, I have heard similar words from caregivers and families all too often. How can any of us understand, if we have not had to personally care for a person who has Alzheimer's disease? How can we even try to help others, if we do not understand?

Take the example of one patient whose wife brought him into a medical studies office for pre-testing. He had been a most successful and enterprising entrepreneur in his northern hometown. He was so successful that he and his wife could retire at an early age, build a spacious waterfront home on a southwest Florida island shore, and enjoy the rest of their lives together, or so they thought. They never anticipated anything like the devastation of hearing he had Alzheimer's disease. Fifty-eight years old, youthful appearance with sandy hair and a rugged tan, and he can no longer find his way to his own home! Try to imagine the fear, the anger, the frustration of having a husband with a healthy body, yet knowing his brain cells are being killed off by this dreaded thing called Alzheimer's disease. And there is little you can do to slow the process!

Just imagine being 52 years old, personally witnessing the birth of your first grandchild, and one hour later asking your family why you were visiting your daughter in the hospital. Or put yourself in the place of a 72-year-old grandmother sitting down to write a letter to her eldest son, and not being able to recall his first name as she begins the letter. Yes, occasionally memory lapses happen to all of us. We have many things on our minds. But it is when these episodes of memory loss compound and interfere with normal daily activities, that families begin to fear the dreaded diagnosis of probable Alzheimer's disease.

One caregiving spouse explained it this way:

"Alzheimer's is the most devastating disease for the family of anyone who has it. Other diseases may be harder on the patient, but nothing can compare to the effect of Alzheimer's on the patient's family. It has been called 'the long good-bye' among other things. It can last from a few years to as many as 20 years or more. Caregivers watch their loved ones deteriorate and regress back to infancy, eventually with no memory at all. It is as if the person you loved is no longer there. Actually, what you are caring for at the end is a physical body."

People who have cared for a loved one with Alzheimer's disease want to speak out on behalf of those loved ones. They want others to know what it is like, so that together we can begin to understand and help one another. Caregivers have formed support groups throughout the world. They get caring support from talking with one another about the perils of having a loved one with Alzheimer's disease. They learn ways to cope. They learn new ideas for care. And, they all seem to have the desire to SPEAK OUT. This book offers them an opportunity to tell all of us about their feelings as caregivers of persons with Alzheimer's disease.

The first three chapters of my book will consist of information, facts, and findings about Alzheimer's as the disease. The subsequent chapters were, in essence, "written" by those who responded to a survey asking "What do you wish others knew and understood about Alzheimer's disease?"

I have compiled within this publication the responses to my surveys from over 200 caregivers. I personally thank each and every one of them who took the time to share their heartfelt stories and their personal feelings. Their courage to speak out and their determination to help others will benefit all of us: family, friend, student and professional alike. Together we can begin to understand and learn new ways to cope and care for persons with this dementing disease, because we are learning from the finest teachers, the experienced—the caregivers of those afflicted with Alzheimer's disease.

1
THIS DISEASE
CALLED ALZHEIMER'S

Alzheimer's disease (pronounced Alz'-hī-merz or Allz'-hī-merz) is a progressive, degenerative disease that attacks the brain and results in impaired memory, thinking and behavior. It is the most common form of dementia, with four million Americans estimated to have the disease. Nineteen million Americans say they have a family member with Alzheimer's disease, and 37 million Americans *know* someone with the disease. Most of these people are asking the same questions: Is Alzheimer's disease the same as dementia? Didn't we use to call it "senility" or "hardening of the arteries?" Isn't memory loss normal as we age?

Dementia describes a brain disorder in which the loss of intellectual abilities is sufficient enough to hinder social and occupational functioning so severely that it interferes with an individual's normal existence. However, dementia can be caused from various brain disorders. If your doctor has told you that your loved one has "dementia," you may want to find out the exact cause of the dementia. Fifty-five percent of all dementia is caused by Alzheimer's disease. Twenty to 30 percent is caused by strokes, and 10 to 20 percent by other causes, many of which are treatable. That is why an early diagnosis to determine the cause of symptoms, such as repetitive memory loss and personality changes, is so important. Diet or medications may also play an important part in memory loss, disorientation and confusion symptoms. Alzheimer's disease is a primary degenerative dementia: a loss of brain cells, neuro connectors, and neuro transmitters, for which there is no cure or current treatment to halt the disease progression. The disease affects a person mentally, emotionally, and physically. It eventually causes death.

More and more people are recognizing their own symptoms earlier, and with early diagnoses, are becoming much more aware of their own disease. In the past, most dementing behavior of the elderly was referred to as "senility," and these elderly persons were sent to nursing homes, often prematurely. Knowing that only an autopsy can give a 100-percent-accurate determination of Alzheimer's disease, new specific testing is increasingly leading to an earlier probable diagnosis long before a person is incompetent or in need of full care.

The clinical course this disease takes in each individual has some similarities, but the symptoms vary so greatly, it is difficult to place any time lines on the deterioration. It seems the younger a person is when diagnosed with Alzheimer's disease, the faster he/she deteriorates. Yet the deterioration is not like a stroke, where memory loss and personality changes occur almost instantaneously. Alzheimer's disease begins with gradual deterioration and continues on a long path of degeneration often lasting 10 to 12 years.

Alzheimer's disease can be better understood in definition through identifying symptoms in three stages: early, middle and late-stage Alzheimer's. In the early stages, lasting approximately two to four years even prior to the diagnosis, short-term memory loss begins to affect work and daily living activities. Often confusion becomes apparent, even with the most mundane, familiar tasks. A person will become lost, even in familiar surroundings. This early stage sometimes manifests itself in mood and personality changes resulting in little initiative, no spontaneity, or a lack of zest for life. Poor judgment can compound the problems, making even routine chores and tasks difficult. That explains why people in the early stages of Alzheimer's disease often have trouble handling money or paying bills. In addition, they seem to lose things constantly and often blame others of "stealing" from them.

This first stage is the phase in which the person is still competent to make a will and to understand it. This is the time to make decisions about care to legally and financially prepare for the future in a realistic way. This is why an early diagnosis is so important.

The middle or second stage is the longest stage, often spanning two to 10 years in time. During this phase, increasing memory loss and confusion may make it necessary to provide full-time supervision to otherwise healthy, active individuals. Their attention span becomes shortened, and they often appear restless and pace or wander endlessly. They frequently repeat statements or even movements, over and over. Occasionally they have repetitive twitches or muscle jerking. This stage is very difficult because problems recognizing family members and close friends become apparent. Individuals with Alzheimer's disease have difficulty organizing their thoughts or even thinking logically. Word recall can become difficult and they may make up words to replace real words. They may have problems with reading or writing, or understanding numbers. Sometimes they develop fears and suspicions, or even see or hear things that are not there. They may even develop a fear of dressing or bathing because they misunderstand these concepts of daily living. Some lose weight and others gain weight during this period.

The third and final stage of Alzheimer's disease is the terminal phase. Alzheimer's disease is a fatal illness. There is no known cure as of this writing. This end stage is usually the shortest phase, yet emotionally, for a family, can seem like the longest, most difficult stage of all. During this phase there is little recognition of self or family. Most people lose weight because of difficulty swallowing. There is little or no capacity remaining to care for one's self. Most communicate very little or not at all. Bladder and bowel control become a problem, and many develop skin infections. Some have seizures and most sleep more. When awake, many groan or scream, put things in their mouth or suck on everything in sight. They need help in every phase of their daily living skills including bathing, dressing, eating and toileting.

The best care management, and the *only* approach that works for Alzheimer's patients in these final two phases, is lots and lots of tender loving care (TLC). A TLC plan begins with understanding this disease called Alzheimer's and learning from the many caregivers who, through their years of trial and error, teach others about care. There are few Alzheimer's textbooks or curricula for doctors and nurses to learn about the treatment and care. Alzheimer's care was not a part of most college curricula. Most have learned from the caregivers, and today they continue to learn new approaches through trial-and-error, trial-and-success, research, and especially from the experiences of others who care for Alzheimer's patients.

The daily practical management of a person with Alzheimer's disease is the key to successful care. It is advisable for a family to pick one "chief,"– one who knows everything about the care management of that patient. As a team of family members and professional service providers, it is up to each individual to learn all you can about home and community resources together. As a "seasoned" or experienced caregiver, *share* all you are able about the resources, ideas and communication skills you have developed.

In the subsequent chapters readers will have an opportunity to not only experience the events in caring for persons with Alzheimer's disease, but they will also have an opportunity to learn from such sharings. Learning from others' experiences will give readers the ability to recognize, understand, and anticipate behaviors and the appropriate responses. Whether it be a family member, a close friend, a neighbor or a patient who has Alzheimer's disease, they and their caregivers need friendship and support – and understanding. With four million afflicted persons in the United States today, everyone will know someone who has Alzheimer's disease. Education is the key to helping others who are struggling with the devastation of this cruel disease.

☥

2
RESEARCH:
WHAT WE ARE LEARNING ABOUT
ALZHEIMER'S DISEASE

Even though Alzheimer's disease was identified and documented over ninety years ago, it has only been in the past 20 years that this disease has been studied, used more frequently as a diagnosis, and received research funding. It has only been in the very recent past that Alzheimer's disease has received valuable media attention, thanks to former President Ronald Reagan.

Historical data reveals that in 1906, Dr. Alois Alzheimer, the German neurologist, had been treating a young, 51-year-old female patient who showed all the signs of severe senility: memory loss, disorientation, and hallucinations. After the patient's death, Dr. Alzheimer examined her brain and discovered areas of clumps of neurofibrillary tangles and groups of plaque. For the next 60 years, physicians thought the condition to be rare and called it "pre-senile dementia." But in the 1960's, researchers found the exact same type of "tangles" in elderly patients and concluded it was not just an abnormality of younger people; it occurred far more frequently than previously believed.

Brain Changes

Two principal changes in the brain tissue of a person who has Alzheimer's disease are "neuritic plaques" and "neurofibrillary tangles." Neuritic plaques are chemical deposits consisting of degenerating nerve cells combined with a form of protein called beta amyloid. Neurofibrillary tangles is the name given to malformations within nerve cells. Although not visible through a CT scan or MRI, the brains of Alzheimer's patients of all ages reveal such changes upon an autopsy examination.

Causes

The causes of Alzheimer's disease are still not known, but they are currently receiving intensive scientific investigation. New break-through information is shared each day, providing a mere piece of the Alzheimer's disease "puzzle" or mystery. Suspected causes being investigated include diseased genes or a genetic predisposition, abnormal protein buildup in the brain, and environmental toxins. The following information will provide some insight into current research findings.

Alzheimer's Disease Associated Protein (ADAP)

Research has discovered a protein called Alzheimer's Disease Associated Protein (ADAP) in the autopsied brains of Alzheimer's patients. This protein, which seems to appear only in people with Alzheimer's disease, is mainly concentrated in the cortex covering the front and side sections of the brain, regions involved in memory function. Researchers have found ADAP not only in brain tissue, but also in the spinal fluid. If they can perfect a test to detect the protein in the cerebrospinal fluid, or potentially even circulation in the blood, it may be possible to use this method of diagnosis on living patients. For now most professionals agree, "Alzheimer's disease is the most overdiagnosed and misdiagnosed disorder of mental functioning in older adults."

Dr. Rudy Tanzi, Director of the Genetics and Aging Unit, Massachusetts General Hospital, was instrumental in helping to discover the first of the known familial Alzheimer's disease genes in 1987, called the amyloid beta protein precursor. There appeared to be a connection with this gene and the Downs Syndrome gene. Dr. Tanzi reports, "The connection between Alzheimer's disease and Downs Syndrome is that the APP gene resides on chromosome 21, the same gene in which persons with Downs Syndrome have three (instead of the normal two) chromosomes." Dr. Tanzi reports that she began researching Alzheimer's disease in 1983 by first researching Downs Syndrome. "I then became intrigued as to why individuals develop Alzheimer's disease pathologicity in the brain, and that led me to discover the first Alzheimer's disease gene."

Much is being learned, especially in the last two decades, about the clinical process of Alzheimer's disease. Both lay persons and professionals are benefiting from the new knowledge and applying this information to appropriate and proper care of persons with Alzheimer's. It is imperative for caregivers to become aware of the newest studies, yet understanding that results are *studies*, not conclusions, about Alzheimer's disease.

In mid-1997, the Alzheimer's Disease Center at the University of Pennsylvania published their findings in the July issue of the *American Journal of Pathology* which stated that lesions made of a previously unidentified protein have been found in the brains of Alzheimer's patients. This discovery could shed light on the cause of the disease and offer a means of early diagnosis and treatment of Alzheimer's disease. Unlike the plaque that Dr. Alzheimer described in 1907, the University team found new lesions made of different material. "It occupies as much of the Alzheimer's brain as amyloid plaques do," the researchers concluded. "As a result, we have every reason to suspect that this pathology will be found to play a crucial role in the development and progression of Alzheimer's disease."

Diagnostic Testing

Many people were hopeful recently when the news about pupillary dilatation tests with Tropicamide showed significant value in determining the existence of Alzheimer's disease in the brain. Although studies are continuing, at this time pupillary dilatation has not been shown to be a reliable test for the presence of Alzheimer's disease. Other diagnostic procedures like spinal fluid TAU capital protein is 80 percent predictive of Alzheimer's disease, and SPECT scanning shows 73 percent accuracy. Some physicians use MRI scans to measure the volume of the hippocampus, which is the short-term memory center of the brain. This has been a possible indicator of Alzheimer's disease, but again, not 100 percent accurate. Even with the discovery of the Apo E4 gene as the contributory factor in Alzheimer's disease, the test for its presence only really shows an increased predisposition of the disease, not necessarily an accurate prediction.

Preventative Measures

Ibuprofen and other nonsteroidal anti-inflammatory drugs (NSAID) have recently been in the news because studies are showing that they may reduce the risk for developing Alzheimer's disease. The Alzheimer's Association says that these results suggest that analgesics may one day play a role in delaying the onset and possibly preventing Alzheimer's disease. However, although very encouraged by the preliminary findings, the Alzheimer's Association also cautions against the use of NSAIDs until further testing is completed.

In January, 1997, Dutch and Belgian researchers reported they found clear evidence linking Alzheimer's disease with clogged arteries. They said Alzheimer's patients were more likely to have atherosclerosis, which is fat clogging the arteries. They also said a blood protein known as apolipoprotein-E played a strong role. Doctors said this is not surprising, as atherosclerosis can reduce blood flow to the brain

Vitamin E and Alzheimer's Disease

Ordinary Vitamin E pills are showing some promise in moderately slowing Alzheimer's disease in patients with moderately severe symptoms who took high doses of it in a two-year study. Actually, Vitamin E was said to have the same effect as the more costly drug called Eldepryl (seligiline), a prescription drug for Parkinson's disease, that also slowed the Alzheimer's disease process. Both Vitamin E and seligiline showed promise in decreasing Alzheimer's disease patients' loss of ability to bathe, dress, handle money and do other routine tasks. Patients who were taking higher doses of Vitamin E scored better in these activities of daily living in about 25 percent of the cases studied. Again, additional studies must be done. Some doctors, however, are routinely recommending Vitamin E to their patients with Alzheimer's disease, and seeing promising results.

Estrogen Replacement Therapy

Recent studies have indicated that the use of estrogen in hormone replacement therapy seems to delay the symptoms of Alzheimer's disease. The largest such study available shows estrogen replacement therapy among postmenopausal women lowers the risk of developing Alzheimer's disease by more than 50 percent. The results of this study, which monitored 472 women over a 16-year period, were detailed in the *Journal of Neurology* in the summer of 1997. This study is not only the first long-term analysis of the effects of estrogen on Alzheimer's disease, but it also is the latest in a series of reports showing the potential for estrogen therapy as an alternate treatment for Alzheimer's disease.

"This is a much-needed confirmation of earlier studies," states the Alzheimer's Association. They caution women, however, not to begin using estrogen solely to protect themselves against Alzheimer's disease: "Further studies need to be completed to test the long-term side effects and resulting memory enhancement theories."

Small Strokes and Alzheimer's Disease

In March, 1997, University of Kentucky scientists reported in the *Journal of the American Medical Association* that preventing small strokes could dramatically reduce the risk of developing the symptoms of

Alzheimer's disease. Their findings appear to solve a long-standing mystery of why many people, whose brains are riddled with the tell-tale dead spaces of Alzheimer's disease, never suffer from the memory loss and physical deterioration marking the disease. In the study, autopsies were performed on the brains of 61 nuns who showed the typical plaques and tangles of Alzheimer's disease. The nuns who suffered small strokes in critical brain areas were nearly twice as likely to have symptoms of Alzheimer's when they were alive. The findings suggest that when a brain is already weakened by Alzheimer's disease, the additional damage caused by a small stroke is enough to precipitate memory problems, as stated by David A. Stone, epidemiologist at the University of Kentucky.

In March, 1997, the *Journal of the American Medical Association* devoted a special issue to Alzheimer's disease research. They cited research on early detection, how small strokes in specific regions of the brain dramatically increase the risk of Alzheimer's disease, and a new formula to help physicians estimate the amount of time before an Alzheimer's patient requires full-time care, or dies. It appears scientists are a long way from controlling Alzheimer's disease, even with the accelerated research. Sadly, "There is not much to offer today's patients in the way of prevention or cure," says the National Institute of Aging.

New Medications

The truth of the matter is this: even though Alzheimer's was identified as a dementing illness ninety years ago, little was found in research or explanation about this disease until the last twenty years. Since it takes 10 to 12 years to complete the clinical trials of new drugs in the United States, it is understandable why there are so few drugs to treat or slow the process of Alzheimer's disease today. When a family discovers a loved one has Alzheimer's, many naturally want to know what medication will eradicate this disease. They assume that there must be *something* that can be prescribed for Alzheimer's disease.

Many health professionals, as well as the general public, are angry to think the medical profession spent the past 90 years developing surgical procedures and medications to allow people to live to be 100 years old, but did so very little to anticipate the brain deterioration. New drugs to slow the dementing process of Alzheimer's disease are being studied. There is still no cure; it is not known what causes this fatal brain disease.

When researchers began addressing the treatment of Alzheimer's disease, their primary goal was to find a drug to manage or prevent Alzheimer's disease, improve cognitive symptoms, slow or stop the progression of the disease, delay the onset of symptoms, and finally, to develop a drug to prevent the disease altogether. The first drug approved to slow the process of the disease was Tacrine. In the early 1990's, the approval of Tacrine (also known as Cognex) specifically for the treatment of Alzheimer's disease, thrust drug development into a brand new era. Tacrine was the first drug approved in the United States for the treatment of Alzheimer's disease. This drug proved to be a costly venture and most people had unavoidable side effects which resulted in the discontinuation of their medication.

One of the greatest costs of taking Tacrine is the weekly blood work needed to assure the liver is not getting damaged from this drug. Those who can tolerate Tacrine, and tolerate it at higher dosages, do very well during certain stages of the disease. However, even today, most people cannot tolerate this drug.

A new drug named Donepezil (also called Aricept) came on the market in late 1996. Aricept was designed specifically for the treatment of mild to moderate Alzheimer's disease. It is chemically unrelated to Tacrine and therefore is well-tolerated without costly liver function testing for side effects. This medication enhances cognitive functioning, hopefully delaying the symptoms associated with memory loss. It has been shown to double the time Alzheimer's victims are able to perform and maintain their own activities of daily living. As a once-a-day dose, it is convenient and easy to administer and use, and it produces cognitive improvement in a majority of patients. In the clinical trials, 82 percent of the patients treated with Aricept experienced improvement in cognition, or no further deterioration in cognition, while on the new medication.

Research companies are working feverishly to find medications to stall the progression of Alzheimer's disease. Many are also making their discoveries available to the many people in need. The Pfizer and Eisai corporations have even developed the Aricept Patient Assistance Program for those United States residents without prescription drug coverage through either public or private insurance, and who fall within certain income criteria. In addition, they have developed a computer database called the "Community Resources for Alzheimer's Disease" to help identify federal, state, and local programs that may provide services to the elderly and/or patients with Alzheimer's disease and their families. This program is available to patients through their physicians' offices.

Many studies continue for drugs which will maintain the cognitive functioning for those with Alzheimer's disease. Two new drugs, Exelon-3300 and Metrifonate, show very promising benefits and are likely to be released within the next few years. With these two new drugs, physicians and families will have four drug-treatment options to choose from for maximum results: to slow the process of brain deterioration.

Social Research Studies

Social researchers examine the treatment and care of Alzheimer's patients, as well as care facilities, to try to scientifically measure outcomes of patient care and behavior under various conditions. Some units are being specifically designed to meet the care needs of clients with Alzheimer's disease by using specific architectural cues and design features to prompt residents' memory. Researchers are examining architectural structures, care procedures, and behavior outcomes to gain important information to enhance the care of those with Alzheimer's disease.

Conclusion

All of the latest findings in Alzheimer's disease diagnosis and treatment offer encouraging new hope for Alzheimer's victims and their families. Alzheimer's disease is becoming a dementia with *some* identifiable brain pathology and treatment at multiple levels. Alzheimer's disease is now considered a diagnosable and treatable condition, and continuing research will result in better diagnoses and the potential for cures for this condition.

Many studies: physical, psychological and social, continue to be conducted in a desperate attempt to identify, understand, and cure Alzheimer's disease. For now, we rely on the experience of caregivers, who teach us through the sharing of their personal experiences, how to understand and treat a person with Alzheimer's disease. The resulting chapters of this book relay caregiver "research" information and findings, in their own words, through their own "studies.".

3
FACTS ABOUT ALZHEIMER'S DISEASE AND CAREGIVERS

"Alzheimer's Disease" was first described by Dr. Alois Alzheimer in 1906. Since then, researchers have developed a deeper understanding of the changes in the brain that occur with Alzheimer's disease. They can identify plaques and tangles in the brain, which, together with behavior changes, characterize the disease. In addition, they are beginning to identify major risks factors such as age and familial history.

The diagnosis itself for Alzheimer's disease remains difficult, although modern medical specialists are getting closer to identifying and diagnosing Alzheimer's disease earlier and with more accuracy. The truth is that a brain biopsy, conducted at an autopsy, is the only way to *positively* diagnose Alzheimer's disease. Through a process of elimination of other causes, the diagnosis of "dementia of the Alzheimer's type" or "probable Alzheimer's disease" is the given diagnosis.

A series of physical and psychological tests are often conducted to properly identify Alzheimer's disease and to help rule out other causes of dementia. Sometimes the same symptoms of memory loss, behavior changes, and disorientation are caused by depressive disorders, head trauma, brain tumors, thyroid or liver problems, infections such as syphilis, Vitamin B12 or Thiamin deficiencies, lupus, or medications themselves. That is why testing by a specialist is the most important source for identifying the cause of the dementia symptoms. "Picks disease" is another variation of dementia that mimics the symptoms of Alzheimer's disease. It has a slightly different pathological outcome however, and so has been separately identified.

The United States Department of Elder Affairs estimates that 17 percent of the population over 65 years of age now has dementia. Forty-seven percent of the population over the age of 85 has dementia. Four million people in America have Alzheimer's disease and that number will triple by the year 2050 if the cause and treatment are not identified. Mental decline which often signals Alzheimer's disease can begin at any age. Alzheimer's is a fatal disease. In fact, Alzheimer's is the fourth leading cause of death in the United States today.

Normal changes in the brain during the aging process include brain atrophy which is a decrease in the size of the brain. At age 20, the average brain weighs about 3.1 pounds. The normal brain of a 70-year-old weighs about 2.6 pounds. The average brain of an elderly person with Alzheimer's disease, however, is 2.0 pounds, a 30 percent decline in size and weight. There is a normal decrease in brain size along with a mild decrease in the cerebral blood flow to the brain as one ages. This results in normal EEG changes on brain wave tests and some impairment of speed on performance tasks. Most people do retain their verbal skills, personality, and social skills as they age without Alzheimer's disease.

In 1997 the U.S. Department of Elder Affairs released these staggering facts about Alzheimer's disease:

- 1 in 5 persons over the age of 65 can expect to develop Alzheimer's disease.
- 1 in 2 persons over the age of 85 has Alzheimer's disease.
- Two times as many women as men living today have Alzheimer's disease, but this is based on the fact that women live longer than men. Percentage-wise, Alzheimer's disease affects both men and women equally.
- Alzheimer's disease affects the same percentage of people worldwide. Every industrialized country struggles with the causes and cures for this devastating disease.

❡

According to census demographics, the elderly population is one of the most rapidly growing segments of our society today. Each day 5,600 people celebrate their 65th birthday. Most Americans living today will reach the age of 85 and beyond. It is estimated that the American *elderly* population will grow from 33 million to an estimated 53 million in the next 25 years, a 61 percent increase. In the state of Florida, the fastest growing population segment is the 100-plus age group, followed by the 85-plus age group. With increasing age comes the higher potential for developing Alzheimer's disease. With the over-85 age group increasing every year, who is going to take care of all the people who are approaching 90? Baby-boomers are facing these questions now as they care for their elderly parents and worry about their own future as they themselves age.

Recent studies by the Alzheimer's Association revealed these facts and figures about those with Alzheimer's disease:

- An estimated 5.8 million Americans over the age of 65 will have Alzheimer's disease in 10 years.
- If no cure is discovered, an estimated 14 million Americans will have Alzheimer's disease by the year 2050.
- Alzheimer's disease is the fourth leading cause of death in adults, after heart disease, cancer and stroke.
- The rate of progression of Alzheimer's disease varies from person to person, with the time from the onset of symptoms until death ranging from 3 to 20 years.
- The average life span after diagnosis of Alzheimer's disease is about 8 years.

Who are the caregivers for all of the people with Alzheimer's disease today? In September, 1996, the Alzheimer Association released the results of a survey of 500 caregivers conducted by Yankelovish Partners, Inc. Their survey results revealed these facts:

- An estimated 70% of the four million Americans with Alzheimer's disease are cared for at home.
- Most caregivers are adult children or spouses who spend an average of 69-100 hours per week caring for their loved ones, the time depending on where the person with Alzheimer's disease resides.
- On the average, the caregivers surveyed are in their mid-fifties and have a median annual household income of $35,000.

Survey results identified caregivers of loved ones with Alzheimer's disease with these statistics:

- 81% of caregivers are women
- 50% of all caregivers live with their loved ones, making theirs a 24-hour-a-day job
- 30% are sole caregivers with no outside help
- 96% said caring for loved ones with Alzheimer's disease is "a labor of love"

Further questioning of caregivers revealed these facts:

- nearly 80% of caregivers report high levels of stress- induced psychological and physical ailments
- 90% said it was "frustrating"
- 87% said it was "draining"
- 87% said it was "painful"
- 75% said they are depressed, at least occasionally
- 45% feel they are not getting enough sleep
- 49% strongly agreed their caregiving duties "cause stress within my family"
- 49% agree with the statement: "I do not have enough time for myself"

✗

- 34% fear they will not be able to continue caring for their loved one much longer
- 34% of caregivers of persons in middle to late-stage Alzheimer's are depressed most of the time

The Alzheimer's Association reports the cost of caregiving can cause major financial burdens for some families. Caregivers responding to financial questions answered in this way:
- 59% of caregivers contribute part of their personal income/savings to pay for the care of a loved one with Alzheimer's disease.
- 54% are concerned about how they will continue to pay for the care of their loved ones.
- 49% of caregivers report they made financial sacrifices to care for loved one.
- 36% had to reduce their working hours to do the caregiving
- 36% report a loss of income due to caregiving responsibilities
- 35% report being less effective at work because of caregiving responsibilities.
- 31% of family caregivers for persons with severe Alzheimer's report their finances have been "greatly affected" by their caregiving responsibilities.
- 20% have had to stop working primarily to care for a loved one with Alzheimer's disease.
- 13% were turned down for a promotion because of their caregiving responsibilities.
All of these financial considerations result in 64% of family caregivers saying they are concerned about having enough money to take care of their own needs as they grow older.

The survey revealed that most caregivers are generally realistic about a loved one's prognosis:

- 81% strongly agreed Alzheimer's disease is a progressive, deteriorating disease.
- 63% do not expect a cure for Alzheimer's disease during a loved one's lifetime.
- 77% said they would be happy if medications being developed to treat Alzheimer's disease could stabilize the progression of a loved one's condition.

In another study conducted by the Department of Elder Affairs, these findings were reported:
- 86 % of elder Americans want to remain independent and live out their lives at home in the company of family and friends.
- 90% of caregivers work outside the home in addition to caring for loved ones.
- About one-third of all caregivers missed a month or more of work during their entire caregiving experience.
- An estimated 50% of caregivers are suffering from burn-out.

According to the Alzheimer's Association survey, those with a loved one in a nursing home or other assisted-living facility are more likely to be depressed than caregivers whose loved ones reside on their own, or with the caregiver, friends or family members. More than anything else, caregivers in this survey reported a need for someone to share the burdens of care from time to time. Of those who reported this need:
- 28% preferred home health care
- 10% preferred respite care through a temporary nursing home
- 7% preferred respite through adult day care

It is these staggering facts that led this author to the task of writing this book. Caregivers need to share the burden of care, if not through direct help, than through the understanding of family, friends, and professionals. Caregivers need optimism; they need hope for a future that will bring about awareness of the perils of Alzheimer's disease. They need to be able to speak out to the press, to the government, to the professionals, and to researchers about this devastating disease that has wreaked havoc for themselves and their families. They need to tell anyone who will listen.

The following chapters will help validate the above statistics, giving caregivers an opportunity to share their views, in their own words.

4
IN THE BEGINNING:
OBSERVATIONS AND COVER-UPS

The earliest symptoms of Alzheimer's disease may reveal itself through a gradual deterioration of one's memory, especially short-term memory, and abnormal, inconsistent behavior patterns and personality changes. Additional symptoms of Alzheimer's disease may include decline in the ability to perform routine tasks, disorientation, difficulty in learning new material, and loss of language skills. Some people cover up their symptoms by joking about it, or gradually withdrawing from social affairs for fear of family or friends noticing their memory decline. They often fear they will be ridiculed by their friends for repeating stories and questions, and so they choose to disengage themselves from normal activities. Often married couples begin to experience severe difficulty in communicating, as the well-spouse corrects and contradicts the memory blunders of the spouse with beginning Alzheimer's disease symptoms. Many parents can fool their adult children who live a distance away into believing everything is just fine. Most often the real symptoms are not identified as symptoms of Alzheimer's disease until years later, when a family can look back in retrospect and see the progression of the disease.

A recent study revealed about one in five families with someone suffering from Alzheimer's disease fails to recognize the symptoms of the disease for many years. As a result, many Alzheimer's patients miss their last opportunities to fully participate in planning their own long-term care or family financial future. Many participants in this survey commented on what it was like "in the beginning." The earliest symptoms were often missed or denied as symptoms of Alzheimer's disease, simply because a family does not believe this could be a true diagnosis. Close family members, as well as the affected individual, are very clever at covering up the disease symptoms. Many family members search their memories to try to identify exactly when they first suspected symptoms of Alzheimer's disease in a loved one Following is what many of them had to say about the early symptoms.

First Impressions and General Observations

Often the subtle changes that take place in the early stages of Alzheimer's disease are overlooked or attributed to other causes. These caregivers recall their first impressions and thoughts:

"He started to forget simple things like his phone number."

"I wish I had known more about the disease in the beginning. There were so many warning signals, but it took us years to identify the cause and then learn to accept the diagnosis."

"The saddest thing was when my father's memory of different things began to fail, and he began wandering and forgetting where he was."

"My knowledge of Alzheimer's was based on friends' accounts of their relatives who had the disease: getting up in the middle of the night; dressing inappropriately; walking outside naked; urinating on the wall, or worse. I really didn't think my mother would ever fall into one of those categories! So her early memory loss symptoms didn't really concern me at first. I was certain that MY Mom was just forgetful!"

"When I first realized it was a possibility that my mother had Alzheimer's, my thought was 'Will I have it, too?'"

"He began to follow me like a shadow," said one spouse about her husband's early symptoms. Often previously independent people cling to a spouse or family member as their disease progresses. Some believe this is a desperate attempt to hold onto reality. Others see it as a terrified

fear of their failing judgment, thus relying on that loved one for help.

Loving spouses, after many years together, most often know their mates better than any one else does. They observe changes many others never see. One devoted spouse explained it this way:

"To an observer, he usually looks good. But I can see the fright in his eyes as his memory fails him. To a casual observer, he appears normal. They have no idea how frightened we both are about his memory loss."

Dr. Franklin Cassel in his booklet "Flowers for Peggy" said this of his spouse:

"As I look back on those years, I believe the problem first showed itself as Peggy lost confidence in finding her way in what had been familiar territory. I recall our having visited someone in the hospital and being surprised, when we were ready to leave, by Peggy's reluctance at my suggestion she meet me at the front entrance where I would bring the car. This we had done many times before. I now realize Peggy was beginning to forget her way about and was ashamed to tell me she was lost."

The symptoms of Alzheimer's disease can begin as early as ages 30 to 40, but they are more usual between 50 and 80 years of age. The gradual onset of memory disturbances, personality changes resulting in behavior problems, as well as social changes in grooming and dressing, are often the first symptoms noticed. Many caregivers shared their comments about those early symptoms.

Inappropriate Dressing

"One of the earliest signs with my mother was that her normally prim-and-proper, well-groomed appearance began to deteriorate," remarks one daughter.

Due to the confusion accompanying the early signs of Alzheimer's disease, persons who were once very orderly in their thinking, and in their grooming, begin to wear soiled or inappropriate clothing. This is often a first sign to adult children that something is wrong with their parents. An occasional slip into sloppy dress behavior is not alarming, but a consistent pattern of deteriorating appearance is certainly a "red flag" warning.

"One of the earliest symptoms to look for, strictly in my opinion," remarks an observant caregiver, *"is when someone starts wearing layers of clothes. The weather has nothing to do with this because they will do it in the summer also. It is not uncommon to see an Alzheimer's patient wearing two or three pairs of underpants. They also tend to get their clothes on wrong side out or backwards."*

Personality and Behavior Changes

"Mom's personality changed drastically. She showed paranoid tendencies and even challenged service people in a hotel for doing their jobs," related an adult child caregiver, revealing another early symptom. This type of paranoid behavior causes so many arguments between the patient and their family members. Unlike any other physical disease in which we search for the symptoms verifying the disease, Alzheimer's disease symptoms are subtle and hidden. Often such paranoid tendencies have been argued and discussed many times before one realizes that perhaps it is a symptom of Alzheimer's disease.

Another caregiver noted memories of her mother-in-law's earliest signs of inappropriate behavior this way:

"My father-in-law did a good job of hiding my mother-in-law's symptoms from the family. Even though we visited them once a week, he would explain away her strange behavior as she was just tired or upset with him. Maybe we were in denial, too. Alzheimer's happens to the 'other people.' One day while I was visiting my mother-in-law (with no one else around), I observed her daily activities. She ate lunch with her hands, put straws into the blinds on the windows,

and to top the day off, she spit spitballs at me through a straw! It was that afternoon with my mother-in-law that I knew we had become the 'other people.' When my father-in-law came home I had a long talk with him and convinced him to take her to a geriatric specialist. The diagnosis was probable Alzheimer's (early onset)."

For one daughter, the seriousness of her mother's symptoms seemed to culminate in one day:

"I first realized Mum had Alzheimer's disease when she kept phoning and telling me that the clouds where full of germs. Then she decided to visit me and got lost. I spent hours looking for her. This marked the start of my endless flow of tears. That day Mum said, 'Don't cry. I'm sorry I'm doing these things. I must just be stupid.' And I cried more."

Two other caregivers expressed their views on personality changes in this way:

"The hardest part was watching the personality changes in the beginning and not knowing what it was."

"When I first saw my father's unprecedented anger and hostility, I realized that his memory was failing. I was very scared for him."

Even young people are very cognizant of the abnormal behavior:

"My grandma couldn't remember important things and got mad at my Mom for really unimportant things."

A teen-ager tells about the early signs of her mother who was 45 when diagnosed:

"She started to make fun of little things she never used to do. Then she started eating M & M's and other junk food and acted like it just didn't matter anymore. She started needing me to come with her whenever she saw people because she forgot who they were and would need to ask me."

"I first realized my Grandmother had Alzheimer's disease," relates another granddaughter, *"when she started refusing to leave her*

home for more than an hour at a time. This was out of character for Grandma. She had always loved attending birthday parties, holiday events, or get-togethers at my parent's home. It became increasingly evident that her security was her home."

A concerned young daughter remembers it this way:

"He started doing very strange things, like walking to town (15 miles away!) instead of driving his car. He would talk in circles and not make any sense. There were several different things that made us suspect that he had Alzheimer's disease, but the doctor kept telling us 'no' because he was 'too young.' He was only 57 years old!"

Memory Loss

One of the difficulties noted in the earliest days before the diagnosis is the unpredictability of the memory loss and behavior changes:

"There are good days and bad days," explains one family member. *"One never knows what to expect or when."*

Another daughter remarks about the early signs of the unpredictable memory loss this way:

"I first realized my Dad had Alzheimer's disease when we found he had been hiding the mail and companies started to call about unpaid bills. Also, he wanted to go fishing in the boat on one day, then he would vehemently refuse to step foot in the boat the very next day. Looking back on it now, I think he feared he would not be able to find his way home."

A confused husband remembers, *"In the earlier stages, sometimes she would inadvertently talk to me like I was someone other than her husband Joe. She would say 'Joe is at the barber' right to me. Or 'I think Joe would like to go to the movies' when I was standing right there."*

Often the first presenting symptoms go virtually unnoticed, and they don't initially alarm a family member into thinking about Alzheimer's disease:

❧

"My Mom is only 54 years old and was recently diagnosed with Alzheimer's disease. Although I knew something was wrong, I never suspected she could possibly have Alzheimer's at her young age. Her earliest symptoms of difficulty with word recall; losing her purse, glasses, or keys all the time; and her handwriting change, never made me think of Alzheimer's disease. She was a professional career woman and I didn't even realize that she could no longer work, read with any comprehension, or even drive! I just don't know how to help her now."

Sometimes the symptoms are dismissed with humor: *"At first there were jokes about my father being an 'absent-minded professor.' He would say he was too busy thinking about weighty matters to remember names or dates or other mundane things. But then he couldn't even tell time."*

Often, it is unbelievable behavior from an adult who had always acted in a mature fashion, that triggers concern:

"He started to throw pots and pans away after he cooked."

"Sometimes he would call me to say that he had lost his black poodle, who always turned out to be right at his side."

"He had memory loss over most matters he used to be able to handle, and his disposition changed dramatically in a short time."

The unpredictability of this disease: this has to be one of the greatest hardships of all. Not only is the disease hard to diagnose, with only behavior changes as a symptom, but once identified, the course differs so vastly from one person to the next.

Confusion With Once-Familiar Tasks

Difficulty with once-routine, familiar tasks, such as with numbers and accounting, appear to be early symptoms which begin to affect the lifestyles of those in the early stages of Alzheimer's disease. One spouse noted:

"He was having more and more difficulty adding and subtracting numbers and keeping a proper balance in his check book. He got so he could no longer reconcile his check book balance with the bank statements."

"My mother cried at McDonald's because when the order came to $3.92, she didn't know if the four one-dollar bills she had was enough. It broke my heart."

"Sometimes he couldn't tell the difference between $5.00 and $500.00. He was practically giving money away," laments a concerned son.

A wife/caregiver relates the changes in her life this way, *"Even though he was an accountant, all financial worries began to be overwhelming for him. I had to take them over one by one. They are mine alone now."*

Frequently an early sign of memory loss is demonstrated with repetitive confusion in performing once-routinely familiar tasks. A professional caregiver/nurse conveys her observations this way:

"Another early signal of possible Alzheimer's disease is that they lose their ability to perform small everyday tasks, such as changing the channel on the TV or programming the microwave for a previously well-known function. Because of the memory loss, they frequently do such things as turning water faucets on, and then walk off and leave them running."

A daughter-in-law, who also happened to be a nurse, relates this story about some of the first symptoms noticed with her loved one:

"My father-in-law was a prominent eye doctor. He was examining my eyes for new glasses. He acted like he couldn't understand what he could do to help me see better. After I left his office, he called my husband and told him that he must take me to a specialist, because he was afraid that I was going blind. I went to another opthamologist and my eyesight was normal for my age and

✖

degree of myopia. We were shocked to realize his incompetence."

"One of the first symptoms I observed was how confused Mom would get when taking a message over the phone," remarks an attentive daughter. *"She would try to write it down, and struggled with the words to make sense of the message. A short time later, she had no recollection of who had called or what the message was."*

Another daughter recalls, *"My mother began to get confused over the date. She had always been on top of that. She began to have anxiety attacks when she wrote a check, repeated herself constantly, asked the same question five times in 20 minutes. Now she obsesses on things."*

"The saddest thing was when my mother-in-law tried to pick up crafts that she used to do routinely," explains a caring family member. *"She sat there one day with everything in her lap and cried because she didn't know how to get started. I tried to show her, but she just couldn't begin to do it. She cried and begged me not to 'put her away' in a home. It broke my heart."*

"One of the first disease symptoms I noticed was Mom's forgetfulness" remarks this caregiver. *"Once she phoned me (I lived several hours away) to tell me how upset she was that my husband and I were not at her home for the wedding of my cousin later in the day. We knew nothing about it! But she insisted that she had talked to me about it weeks before. It was so frustrating for us—and her!"*

Another family relates this story:

"We live in Kentucky and my mother-in-law lived in Wisconsin. She started to call us at all hours of the day and night. We were on her speed dial. She would ask us helplessly where she was, why she was there, and why didn't we take care of her. All the while, she was in her own home of many years. It is heart-breaking!"

The confusion, the cover-ups, the denial, the paranoid behavior—these are all early symptoms of a disease that is slowly creeping into the brain cells of those who have Alzheimer's. There are no apparent physical changes nor definitive blood tests to quickly identify the disease. There is only a myriad of questionable episodes that are dismissed as "incidental" in the beginning.

Confusion in Once-Familiar Places

All too often, the first symptoms of Alzheimer's disease reveal themselves when there is confusion about the present moment. Once-familiar places suddenly become foreign to the person with Alzheimer's disease, causing fear and confusion.

"I first realized my father-in-law had Alzheimer's disease when he was at his own home on Christmas day and asked my mother-in-law to take him 'home,'" explains this family member.

Sharing her panic, a daughter tells of this episode:

"I was terrified when my mother drove down the wrong way on a familiar freeway exit ramp. That was when I first realized that she might have Alzheimer's disease."

"I first realized my Mom had Alzheimer's disease when she started crying in the middle of a store when we were Christmas shopping," tells one daughter. She went on to explain, *"She cried because she couldn't remember why she was there. My heart broke for her—and me."*

Taking persons who have early-stage Alzheimer's disease out of their normal environment may also result in confusion and disorientation. Frequently it is during these trips that a family faces the reality of the memory loss for the first time:

"I remember the time we visited our daughter, like we did every year for fifteen years, and her dad didn't remember ever having been there before," remarks one spouse.

In addition, traveling and staying in a home other than their own can result in confusion that leads to paranoia:

❡

"One night, while we were visiting our son in another city, my husband woke up and insisted that we had to get out of there because we were 'in somebody's home and they weren't home!'" recalls another spouse.

"My husband had always been so efficient at planning trips" shares this spouse. *"In fact, his memory was so good that he could look at a map, plan the route, and never have to refer to the map again! Now simple car trips are confusing and overwhelming to him."*

Another spouse tells this somber story:

"He used to plan the trips and make all the hotel reservations along the route. In fact, he even made all the arrangements for everyone at our club, too. Now I do all of that. Everything changed after the time he went into the hotel to check us in, and then returned to the car saying he couldn't do it. Why? Because he didn't know how many people or how many rooms we needed for just the TWO of us! It really shocked and scared me, but mostly, it saddened me."

"My uncle said it took him three hours to get home from my house (a 20-minute drive), because 'the signs on the highway were changed.'" recalls one nephew. *"At about the same time, he claimed someone had gone into his house, stolen all his clothes and changed the locks on the door."*

Often family members cannot assess the reality of the situation until they physically spend time with their loved one:

"I first realized my mother had Alzheimer's disease symptoms when I took her to visit my two brothers in Pennsylvania and Florida. I lived in California at the time, and I had flown to Indiana to pick her up to travel with me. I realized then just how serious her memory loss and confusion were after I observed her total confusion in those once-familiar places. One month before that, I received a letter from her in which she repeated three paragraphs (almost word for word) and I was puzzled. Then when I saw her in person, and spent some time with her outside of her home, the reality hit me."

Repetitive Questions

Sometimes the early symptoms begin with irritating repetitive questions. Often this is related to an upcoming event of which the person with Alzheimer's has been informed. Their fear of forgetting the upcoming event results in endless questions and is compounded by forgetting having just asked that question.

Many caregivers shared their frustration about the constant repetitive questions regarding an upcoming event:

"I knew he was getting worse when he would keep asking over and over, every few minutes, 'What time are we going?'"

"If I told him that we were expecting company, he would ask me over and over when they were due to arrive. I struggled with <u>not</u> telling him, on the one hand, and <u>telling him too soon,</u> on the other hand."

The perseverance in answering the repetitive questions, and the temptation to totally ignore the questions, present conflict and frustration for many caregivers:

"He is driving me crazy with asking the exact same question over and over again. He gets on one subject and is relentless in asking the same question. It's hard to remain sane and patient when this occurs day in and day out!"

The Cover-Ups

Many caregivers, out of love, concern and/or embarrassment, try to cover-up for a loved one's behavior and inappropriate conversing.

A lonesome spouse put it this way:

"I am sure in the beginning I covered up for him (since I was very talkative and he was a quiet man), so that our friends did not realize the extent of his problem. Now there is little or no speech, and it is a very lonely time for me."

"We used to play cards with our friends every Friday night," another spouse relays. *"At the beginning I would try to cover up for*

her mistakes, but my wife can't remember the rules any more. She even used to be the scorekeeper, but then she had a problem with that, too. Our friends didn't understand. They ridiculed her. They avoid us now. I miss them."

Another spouse tells exactly why he uses a cover-up to hide his own true feelings: *"We all put on a very brave front for fear of losing friends with our complaints."*

In summary, this family member helps to put these feelings in perspective:

"My father-in-law explained to me that mental illness (as he sees Alzheimer's) is something to be hidden. 'Do not let the world in to see the defects,' he would say. This is how he had been brought up to believe. It took a long time for him to accept the fact that it is OK for people to know that Mom has Alzheimer's disease , and it's OK to ask for help."

Caregiver Regrets

Using cover-ups and denying the real problems may be later reviewed with regret and sadness because of missed opportunities:

"My mother could hide the problem so skillfully that we missed the window of opportunity to talk with her about it," laments a son as he looks back.

Many family members also bemoan the fact that they ignored the earlier symptoms:

"Looking back, now I wish we would have included my Mom more in our discussions about her Alzheimer's disease when she was in the early stages," states this daughter. *"In my mother's case, we never did this. I think we were all too afraid to bring it up to her and now I think that was a big mistake. In fact, I believe it caused a communication problem that still exists today. No one wanted to*

talk to her about it and I believe in the early stages, she must have felt resentment for being left out when she knew we were discussing something about her. What I wouldn't give now to have spoken to her about her desires and fears when she was still able to talk—and think."

"I should have talked more with my father when he could still talk," remarks this daughter. *"I wish I had known early on that he was showing the early signs, but it was swept under the rug and denied."*

A family caregiver expresses it this way:

"I wish from the time of my Dad's first symptoms that we had been more informed that he had this damn disease and what we should do about it right away. There should be a schedule and a checklist handed to the patient and their families upon diagnosis. Also my Dad, who is 84 years old, calls the disease a death sentence. We all have one, but few of us get as long a reprieve as he got. We had talked about his 'short memory' for years. We were not totally surprised when our doctor later confirmed it."

Conclusion

One of the most difficult stages for any family who might have a loved one suffering from memory loss is to ascertain whether their observations reveal possible symptoms of Alzheimer's disease. Because a person with Alzheimer's often seems "normal", realistic fears bring confusion about the necessity to seek a professional opinion. In addition, through denial of the real symptoms, many caregivers hope to postpone an often inevitable diagnosis of Alzheimer's disease.

Early diagnosis, however, can bring some closure to the confusion and can help direct the family into positive action. In the following chapter caregivers share their advice about the need for proper and early diagnosis.

5
THE NEED FOR EVALUATION AND EARLY DIAGNOSIS

There is still no single laboratory test capable of making a 100 percent accurate diagnosis of Alzheimer's disease today. Early and careful evaluation is important, however, because many conditions mimic the symptoms of Alzheimer's disease. Many of these conditions are curable and reversible. Such potentially reversible conditions may include depression, adverse drug reactions, metabolic changes, and/or nutritional deficiencies.

"Alzheimer's disease" as a diagnosis has often been referred to as a "diagnosis by exclusion." A comprehensive evaluation to establish a proper diagnosis for the symptoms should include a careful examination of personal and family health history, physical and neuropsychological exam by a physician, mental status assessment, and other tests including blood and urine, EKG, and chest x-rays and perhaps a CT scan. Today such diagnostic tests can rule out reversible illnesses and determine the presence of Alzheimer's disease within 80-90 percent accuracy.

Diagnostic Testing

Together with physical exams and lab tests, physicians rely on CT scans and neurological exams which include testing mental status, to arrive at a diagnosis of Alzheimer's disease.

The CT (computer-assisted tomography) scan of the brain is done to help establish whether certain other disorders (some reversible), that mimic Alzheimer's disease, are present. Preview of the brain scan results may implicate different causes for abnormal memory loss and personality changes, ruling out Alzheimer's disease.

In the past, forgetfulness was often attributed to "hardening of the arteries." We now know that just sluggish blood flow rarely causes memory loss, but a series of small strokes can. The second most common cause of dementia, after Alzheimer's disease, is multi-infarct dementia. This type of dementia is confirmed by a CT scan or an MRI. Multi-infarct dementia means that several small strokes have caused cells in multiple areas of the brain to die. This type of dementia is more characterized by a sudden and stepwise progressions of memory loss rather than the gradual decline seen in Alzheimer's.

Mental status testing has been an important tool in assessing symptoms and furthering more accurate diagnoses. Common tests used to measure memory/mental status are: the Alzheimer's Disease Assessment Scale (ADAS), the Mini Mental State Exam (MMSE), and the Clinician's Interview-Based Impression of Change (CIBIC). Each has a specific use for assessing cognitive functioning, as well as the changes in mental status.

The ADAS is a clinically-validated scale for measuring cognitive function in those with Alzheimer's disease. The projected decline in ADAS scores for untreated mild to moderate patients is six to twelve points per year. The ADAS, and the more extensive ADAS-cog, examines selected aspects of memory, orientation, reasoning, attention, language, and behavior.

Many health care professionals conduct the MMSE to determine cognition and its changes over time. The MMSE is a 30-point interview which examines orientation to time and place, word recall, language, and attention. The projected decline in MMSE scores for untreated patients is approximately two to four points per year on a 30-point scale.

A CIBIC is a clinician's assessment of change with caregiver input playing a large role. It is a semi-structured subjective instrument intended to examine major areas of patient functioning: general functioning, cognition, behavior, and activities of daily living. It is based on a private interview with caregiver and then with the patient. Many of these diagnostic tools are used during the clinical investigation to determine progression of deterioration.

In 1982, after careful comparative studies into the nature of clinical changes of normal aging and progressive dementia of the Alzheimer's type, a global description of seven major stages of Alzheimer's disease was published. Known as the Global Deterioration Scale (GDS), and published in the *American Journal of Psychiatry*, this research was conducted by Dr. Barry Reisberg and his colleagues. These clinical descriptions have proven very useful in the understanding and description of Alzheimer's disease progression, and they are recognized around the world today. The seven major stages coincide with the stages of infant and child development, but in the reverse order. Stage seven corresponds to a person who needs total care, physically and emotionally, much like an infant to the age of about 18 months. Stage six corresponds to a two to five year old, and progressing down to Stage 4, which parallels an eight to 12 year old, able to live independently, yet requiring family assistance. This new information and knowledge can be instrumental in helping caregivers provide improved care and reduce suffering for patients with Alzheimer's disease.

Although helpful in the awareness of the stages of Alzheimer's disease, Reisberg's scale is merely a "tool" for understanding. It was never meant to be a label of "child developmental age." It is a scale for adults who have this disease, not a child who is maturing. The Reisberg scale is meant as an aid to the improvement in care and treatment of those with Alzheimer's disease to attain the greatest quality and enjoyment of life.

The Need For Early Diagnosis

Researcher Dr. Webster Ross believes a mental status evaluation should be part of a routine physical exam for everyone over 65. In an interesting study he conducted on 191 men with dementia, 21 percent had a primary family caregiver who did not know their family member had a memory problem. Even among men with very severe dementia, 13 percent of family members were unaware of the problem. Dr. Ross estimates that 60 percent of Alzheimer's disease patients develop dementia long before family or doctors notice.

When families miss the early signs of Alzheimer's disease, precious time can be wasted, resulting in the lack of prior planning for care and financial issues. In a recent study at the University of Hawaii (*Journal of the American Medical Association*, March, 1997) researchers emphasized the need for early diagnosis because some dementia also can be prevented or cured.

Another detriment to getting an early diagnosis is that too often physicians are reluctant to give a diagnosis of Alzheimer's disease. Because it is not a positive diagnosis until an autopsy is performed, physicians are hesitant to have that "process of elimination" as their diagnostic conclusion. We are learning from caregivers, however, that a PROBABLE diagnosis can mean so much to helping families prepare for the future.

"He did not actually want to diagnose my father with Alzheimer's, but it would have helped prevent so much grief for us," writes one daughter in retrospect.

A loving wife/caregiver shares from her experience:

"Alzheimer's disease is an illness and nothing of which to be ashamed. It makes it easier when we get a diagnosis and can simply share the fact of the disease with others. When they know what the problem is, it reduces the stress for all concerned. This has all worked very positively for my husband and me."

Understanding the results of diagnostic work-ups of individuals where the question of Alzheimer's disease has been raised can be extremely frustrating to the patient and family alike. One adult son wrote this:

"We were not told that Alzheimer's disease had been specifically diagnosed, but that other possible diagnoses had been dismissed,

leaving Alzheimer's disease as the likely diagnosis by the process of elimination." Unfortunately, this is as honest an answer as physicians can give.

"If caregivers would take the time to document symptoms and behaviors in sort of a diary over time, this could help physicians immensely with a thorough understanding of the person's illness," a physician requested. He submitted this survey response in support of the necessity for early diagnosis and evaluation. He advocates that such evaluations would lead to supportive counseling for both the patient and family in the early stages, and for the staff and caregivers in care facilities as the disease progresses.

An adult daughter urges physicians to assist families with a diagnosis and an acceptance of a diagnosis:

"Physicians need to have practical advice for us about care (where to get help, costs, medicines), to help us set limitations for both the patient and the family. We need to know where to find support groups too. We had none of this at the time we were going through Alzheimer's disease with my Mom."

In turn, a professional caregiver urges families to seek the advice of professionals once the diagnosis is established:

"I wish families would understand that much can be done for patients with Alzheimer's disease through a professional evaluation of the nature and severity of the deficits and evaluation of remaining residual strengths. This would give all caregivers valuable information about the approach and care of the individual."

"When I first heard that my grandmother had Alzheimer's disease, I said 'Thank God!'" remarks a grateful family member. She continues, *"We finally had an answer to a question that had been in my family for years. There was something wrong with my grandmother for five to ten years before she was finally diagnosed. She had even*

been put in a mental hospital after a 'breakdown' of some sort. It was easier to understand her disease with a name on it."

Should the Patient Be Told of an Alzheimer's Diagnosis?

Another question which frequently arises with the early diagnosis is whether to tell a person of the probable diagnosis of Alzheimer's disease, once it is determined. Of course, it depends heavily on the individual, the progression of the disease, and the need to know. Some of those who are diagnosed early are aware enough to desire the honest facts. For others, telling them would serve no useful purpose.

A nurse practitioner who works with the elderly advises:

"If the illness was anything but Alzheimer's disease, I would support wholeheartedly telling the truth to your loved one. However, if your family member with diagnosed Alzheimer's disease cannot remember what you have just said, and reacts with tears, anger, or sadness when you tell him the true diagnosis, then practice good communication skills by validating and distracting. That is, simply tell him that he has a few memory problems, but not to worry because you are there to care for him. And then turn the conversation to another topic."

A volunteer caregiver shared this view:

"I believe patients need to know their own diagnosis as soon as possible. They need to know they are afflicted. It is the humane thing to do. It allows people to get their lives in order, express wishes to their families, and prepare themselves and others for the changes that will occur."

This view was verified through the statement of a person in the early stages of Alzheimer's disease who wrote this:

"I know I have Alzheimer's disease. I can't start a conversation on my own any more. I have been slowly getting worse for about four years. At present I am involved in a drug test for a new drug. I can

still answer some questions when I am asked. I am glad I know my diagnosis. I will do anything to help myself."

An experienced caregiver, however, feels this way:

"It's so important for a family to realize they will never get their loved ones to <u>understand</u> they have Alzheimer's disease. Never, never argue with someone who has Alzheimer's disease to try to <u>convince</u> them of their illness. They no longer have the ability to grasp that concept."

<u>The Importance of Prior Planning</u>

"Tell people to PLAN! Don't get caught in a legal system that can easily 'suck' you dry." This was the warning from several family caregivers, looking back in retrospect. They are urging family members to get that early diagnosis and begin planning for the future of their loved one with Alzheimer's disease just as soon as feasible. *"It can make the difference between financial hardships and wise decisions for a realistic future with your loved one,"* urges one caregiver.

"I wish someone would have told me earlier that there is real urgency to get some things settled as soon as you learn of the diagnosis. My advice to family members: Don't waste precious time arguing about the 'if only's' or 'it can't be's'. Tackle the problems associated with having a family member with Alzheimer's disease as early as possible," implores an experienced caregiver.

Another family caregiver offers this practical advice:

"I want others to know I think the most important thing to do first, after the diagnosis, is to get your loved one to the dentist, eye doctor and hearing specialist as soon as possible. The longer you wait, the more difficult it is to try to overcome the fears and confusion persons with Alzheimer's experience regarding the exams. I'd advise families to get established with such doctors early on so you can get access when needed in the later stages."

No doubt, prior planning will affect the health care industry itself. Since so many individuals have a diagnosis of Alzheimer's disease, it is time for health care to begin planning for the future of these elderly adults who may likely live to be 100 years old. One adult caregiver remarked, *"We need to spend more time training care providers in facilities about dementia behavior and how to interact and care for them and understand their behaviors better."* She continues, *"Many times the person affected is unable to perform what is expected because they have forgotten how to do what is wanted. This makes them inadequate to make decisions about their future. Most of all, we sometimes need help to realize when you cannot give adequate care by yourself any longer and look toward a care facility for help. We need to plan for that inevitable future."*

Another adult caregiver shares this advice:

"My Mom is in the early stages of Alzheimer's disease and I'm learning how to approach everything by talking with other caregivers at weekly support group meetings. I have very little knowledge about the progression of this disease, and I know this is the easy part. I can't imagine how rough it's going to get. So if I can at least get things in the house organized now, and get a semblance of a routine going, I'll be in a better position to handle the later stages."

A spouse/caregiver resolves his advice this way: *"Expect that the unexpected will happen and prepare for it."*

"Get help and counseling while you can," urges another family caregiver. *"You need to be mentally and physically prepared to understand that someone you've known all of your life, who has been strong and independent, will now depend on you for everything. You will end up being responsible for every decision. Yet they will not even remember that you are their son or daughter."*

A nursing professional gives this advice:

"As a nurse, I cannot emphasize enough the need for advance proxy planning for patients with Alzheimer's disease. These patients

become unable to make their own decisions regarding their care. Advance proxy planning is a mechanism for families to protect their loved ones' rights of self-determination. In addition, it gives the caregivers of patients with advanced Alzheimer's the knowledge of the scope of medical interventions to be carried out if certain events occur."

Many hospitals and care centers are adopting advance proxy planning for patients with Alzheimer's disease which resemble the hospice philosophy of care. Even if a patient has a living will, there are usually no exact guidelines regarding specific medical interventions. Advance proxy planning designates a level of care for each patient from aggressive care keeping the patient alive with all medical interventions possible, to limited medical interventions with only supportive care to keep the patient comfortable. The decision regarding the level of care is made at a family conference, with the input of the physician, nurse, patient (if possible) and family together determining the advance proxy plan for future care. *"I encourage all families with a loved one who has Alzheimer's disease to use a family planning meeting as a means to help you together make difficult decisions prior to the immediate need for such decisions,"* states a professional care planner.

Financial and legal matters need almost immediate attention also. Another professional geriatric care manager pleads:

"No matter how early that diagnosis is given, or how young the family member may be, the well-spouse, adult child, or responsible family member needs to seek the help of professional elder law attorneys and financial planners. As difficult as it is to face the fact that your loved one has a dementing brain disease, it is far more difficult to get caught up in legal and financial crises in the future that will drastically limit your choices of care."

Conclusion

The need for early diagnosis and evaluation has clearly been emphasized by family and professional caregivers alike. If the probable diagnosis is Alzheimer's disease, it is up to each family to determine whether a person with Alzheimer's disease should be told of his/her diagnosis, or how planning for the care and needs of that loved one shall proceed. Review the thoughts of those who spoke up about this question and determine what would most compassionately meet the needs of your loved one who has an Alzheimer's disease diagnosis. Consider the wise words of experienced caregivers who have offered suggestions about the necessity for early diagnosis and prior planning.

6

CAREGIVERS SPEAK OUT TO HEALTH CARE PROFESSIONALS

Caregivers conveyed many concerns and frustrations regarding the information, or lack of information, provided by physicians. Some felt their physician ignored their anxieties about initially-observed symptoms. Others sensed a genuine lack of knowledge about Alzheimer's disease on the part of their physicians. Frustration about the insufficiency of physician information, lack of education, and less-than-compassionate support from physicians prompted the following caregiver responses.

"Please Listen to My Concerns"
"The Doctor said, 'Well, she's old; you have to expect memory loss,'" relates one family member who voiced a concern to her physician about changes in her mother's mental capacities. Memory loss is not a normal process of aging. This bears repeating: MEMORY LOSS IS NOT A NORMAL PROCESS OF AGING. Memory loss, however, is not always caused from Alzheimer's disease as learned in the first five chapters of this book. Alzheimer's symptoms can mimic other types of dementia, many of which are reversible, but half of these dementia symptoms are later found to be related to Alzheimer's disease.

Unfortunately, ignoring dementia symptoms and stereotyping of the elderly by professional providers and caregivers is still prominent:

"My doctor tried to reassure me with: 'Your dad is 80 years old,'" remarks another caregiver. *"He told me 'You've got to expect he will be confused and disoriented and suffer from memory loss at his age.' I looked him straight in the eye and begged, 'Please listen to my concerns. This behavior is <u>not</u> normal for my Dad.'"*

❧

It takes audacity to question a physician's judgment call and courage to insist on further investigation into memory loss. Brave caregivers share their frustrations as they seek honest answers, understanding, and support from their physicians.

Many caregivers surveyed expressed their concerns about how long it took for a physician to validate their fears and explore the possibilities of an Alzheimer's disease diagnosis. Various family members, as heard in the previous chapter, felt an earlier diagnosis could have prompted better understanding and helped to avoid many frustrations of waiting, sometimes years, for the "Alzheimer's diagnosis" to finally be spoken. *"It's just old age,"* were frequently the words used by physicians to avoid the recognition of the very real symptoms of this disease.

One daughter expresses her comments this way:

"My doctor's reaction to our concerns about mom's memory loss and personality changes is: 'It's just her age!' I know that's not true! She is only 71! His lack of information and concern is absolutely appalling!!!!! But I am finding out that this is standard. This attitude must change!!!!!!"

"I believe arrogance in some doctors is closely linked to ignorance," this caregiver remarks. *"To have dismissed symptoms of Alzheimer's disease as 'normal aging' only delayed the proper planning and coping we could have had, and replaced it with confusion and arguments."*

"Expect your doctor's ignorance about Alzheimer's disease," states another caregiver, *"but don't accept it. Go to the physician who will properly identify the reasons for the memory loss and confusion. Don't accept it as a normal process of aging."*

A provoked daughter relates this story:

"After my Mom and I returned to her home following a nine-day trip, I was convinced that something was seriously wrong with her memory. I immediately took her to her family doctor. He said

❧

there was nothing wrong. When I pressed on about it perhaps being Alzheimer's, he refused to identify it. After pestering him with many questions, he finally said it did not matter what name or label we give IT, it all means the same. Then he yelled. 'Yes, your Mom has had 'IT' for the last two years!' I was shocked both at his attitude, and the fact that I had not realized that she had Alzheimer's disease that long. I usually only visit her once a year. I asked the doctor about giving her different tests and medications or treatments. The doctor said tests were not necessary and that I had to accept 'IT' because there was nothing we could do about it. Before we left the office, he mentioned that she (Mother) should not be living alone...as it would be dangerous! What would he have said if I had not pressed for a diagnosis or information?!" questions this caregiver in complete frustration.

Feelings of disappointment with her physician were also evident in this caregiver's circumstance:

"When I expressed my concerns to my doctor about my father's memory loss and personality changes, his reaction was like 'zip'— nothing. His only advice was to try to 'medicate' it away! With what?"

Families shared many comments about the seemingly frustrated doctor responses to their inquiries:

"My Dad recently called his physician to get Mom an appointment to discuss her increasing memory loss symptoms," says one daughter, *"and the doctor asked, 'What do you want me to do about it?"*

In addition, doctors' responses can often cause delays in an accurate diagnosis and cause family members to start believing they are fabricating the observed symptoms. This caregiver explains her feelings:

"I noticed Mom began having difficulty taking her anti-convulsing medication, a thing she had been doing four times a day by rote since age 18 (she's 66 now). My doctor referred her to a neurologist who said it was 'normal aging!' GRRRRR! When I finally

got the diagnosis of Alzheimer's disease, there was some relief in that at least there was an explanation. I didn't make it up that something was wrong."

A concerned spouse relates this account:

"My doctor dismissed all of my husband's symptoms by telling us 'everyone forgets!' It took over a year to impress on the doctor there was a real problem. This may have been because he was only 61."

Often when the affected person is younger, physicians reject the psychological symptoms the family conveys. A wife-caregiver vents her frustration:

"I wish doctors were more aware that Alzheimer's affects people who are not that old, and they need to watch for symptoms at earlier ages. Doctors need to be more aware that a person may seem in excellent health, but he may be having unexplained memory problems that his loved one questions, and the doctor dismisses as insignificant. This happened to me and I almost went crazy myself before my doctor listened to my concerns."

"My doctor's comment to me regarding my Mum's diagnosis of Alzheimer's disease was, 'Well, yes, I know your Mother is only 65. So just leave her in her own house until she gets bad enough for long-term care,'" noted one daughter. "He got _his_ when my Mum's drivers' license was canceled due to his report. Mum was so angry at the doctor that each morning for three weeks she attended his surgery and hurled abuse at him until I got a phone call to come and collect her. I drove out there each morning, one hour away, and all I can say is that it was never a _fast_ trip. Is this 'bad enough' for long-term care!"

"Why didn't he tell us?"

Several caregivers vented their anger at physicians who assumed they understood the diagnosis was Alzheimer's disease, when, in fact, they were never told:

"When I first heard the diagnosis, I thought 'Why weren't we told about this years ago?'" questions a young son. *"Her doctor knew; why didn't he tell us? He just assumed that we understood, and the truth is: the diagnosis of Alzheimer's disease never entered my mind."*

Once the diagnosis is known, general lack of available information can lead to further frustration and stress. This caregiver relates her story in retrospect:

"I wish someone would have spent more time with us, educating us about what to expect down the road. Not every family member will have the time to investigate or read the literature about this disease. I will always remember the kind doctor (not my Dad's doctor) who finally sat me down and explained that I needed to start letting go. I needed to do for my dad only the things that would make him comfortable, even if that was only giving him a drink of Ensure. I had been struggling for hours trying to get Dad to eat all the food on his tray. I didn't even know that difficulty swallowing was part of the disease, and I had been forcing my Dad to eat. If only I would have known sooner. I would have avoided a lot of frustration."

"I wish EVERYONE, but especially doctors, understood the most frustrating thing about caring for someone with Alzheimer's disease is the recognition of the problem," argues this family caregiver. She continues, *"Don't allow us and them to go on believing a problem doesn't exist. Case and point: my father-in-law's doctor didn't want to take my father-in-law's driver's license away! So he told Pop it was only a 'temporary' arrangement. I had to get into his face and say it wasn't fair to Pop, giving him false hope when the fact is Pop can no longer drive safely and was always getting lost, even in familiar territory. It's nice that some people want to 'protect' the Alzheimer's patient from reality, but patients also have a right to KNOW. Not knowing and fearing is far worse. I know this from my own personal*

experience with a diagnosis of multiple sclerosis."

"*I wish the medical profession would understand when a parent is first diagnosed with this disease, the adult child is devastated,*" relates another family caregiver. "*I knew my father was getting forgetful and then in a few short months he became severely demented and delusional. I was never told until I had to hospitalize him for psychotic behavior that he had Alzheimer's. I tried to speak with his doctor, but he would not tell me anything. I am the only child and my mother died five years ago. So when I did find out, I had no idea what to do, what it was, or what to expect. I had to do research on my own. Everyone felt like I should just deal with it since he had to go in a nursing home. It is very hard to deal with alone. No one tells you what to say to your parent when he asks questions about things that are delusional or not true. They don't tell you about how your parent will turn against you at first because they have lost control of their lives and have to blame it on someone. It is heart-breaking. I had my Dad at home for five years with me and then, over night it seemed, he got worse and I had to put him in a nursing home.*"

Some adult children bring their parents to a physician for a physical ailment, and then vent their concerns about the psychological changes they are observing. Frequently physicians are more comfortable in treating the physical illnesses:

"*My doctor brushed aside my concerns about Mom's memory loss and personality changes. He was treating her for her thyroid and a cyst on the liver. Since mom was only 64, the doctor thought I was over-reacting. I wish we had gotten our diagnosis of Alzheimer's disease earlier. It would have saved us a lot of heartache.*"

This daughter expresses her thoughts as she recalls her mother's initial doctor visit:

"*My mother's doctor thought she was just being 'an old woman' and would not listen to hers and my complaints about her personality changes and memory loss. Mom is a person for whom I had to pull eye teeth to get to go to the doctor in the first place, so I was relying on his help. He thought we were being worried over nothing. He was wrong!"*

Not all those who answered the survey had negative comments about their physician. When asked who helped them the most in understanding the disease, one daughter/caregiver offered highest praises for her physician:

"My doctor has been great. He has been very helpful and I hope he continues to be!"

"Doctors Don't Have All the Answers"

In addition to the need for better diagnosing, several caregivers vented their disappointment at professionals for their lack of knowledge about treatment, support and referrals. It is important at this point to understand, however, very few physicians had formal training about Alzheimer's disease and its implications on the patient and family. When the majority of current medical people were trained ten, twenty, thirty or forty years ago, "senility" was the only part of dementia in their medical vocabulary. Taber's Cyclopedic Medical Dictionary (1970, page A-59) listed Alzheimer's disease as "presenile dementia which is similar to senile dementia but occurs in the 40-60-year age group". It then briefly added: "the disease has a relentless and irreversible course but may take from a few months to four or five years to go to the stage of complete helplessness." That was the total information given. Today's Taber's devotes a full page to Alzheimer's disease etiology, complete with pictures of the brain and suggested care options.

"We had to learn the hard way that doctors don't have all the answers," concludes a loving elderly spouse who had hoped for a better strategy for her husband's care.

Many families merely get a diagnosis without explanation or referral:

"My physician called it 'presenile dementia.' He knew very little about Alzheimer' diseases."

Some caregivers take that diagnosis and learn all they can:

"I have learned most about Alzheimer's disease from the last six weeks of constant reading and digesting material on this subject. I learned very little from my doctor besides his diagnosis that Mum really had Alzheimer's disease."

Frustrated with his own physician, this caregiver not only sought information on his own, but then shared it with his physician:

"My doctor knew very little about Alzheimer's disease so I did the research until I found the Alzheimer's organization, got a packet sent to me, and gave him copies. This was about 16 years ago."

Another caregiver craves more information:

"I wish the doctor had been more helpful. He didn't seem very knowledgeable. He was understanding, but did not educate me about Alzheimer's disease."

"We need to know from our physicians that there are others in the same or similar situations," urges this caregiver. *"Often we feel so alone."*

One family caregiver offers this suggestion:

"Doctors need to have good information on hand they can give us in writing, so they can refer us to resources locally available and accessible to us."

A concerned daughter comments on the lack of information available to her parents:

"I feel my mother has not gotten enough answers for her to cope well with the changes my father is going through. I think he (the physician) is vague and not too well informed himself about Alzheimer's disease. I wish he had referred them to a gerontologist or someone who had more information."

Oftentimes various diagnoses are given prior to reaching the basic cause of the dementia:

"My mother had a stroke in May of 1991, and was then diagnosed with multi-infarct dementia. One doctor said she had paranoid schizophrenia, and I questioned this diagnosis. It took two and a half years to get the true diagnoses of Alzheimer's," relates a frustrated caregiver. *"Even now her doctors still refuse to actually call it 'Alzheimer's.' The diagnosis is usually 'Dementia of the Alzheimer's Type.' They say there are over four million Alzheimer's patients in the U.S. now, but if they refuse to diagnose it, (I wonder) what is the real number?"*

"There were genetic factors in my mother's condition that her doctor never asked us about," comments another concerned family member. *"My family might have been able to help her through much of the earlier stages had we been prompted by the physician to become aware of what was occurring."*

Various caregivers questioned the rationality of physicians' using normal verbal inquiries to obtain information from a person suffering from memory loss:

"Don't doctors know how to communicate with a person with Alzheimer's disease? Case and point: the Doctor asked my mother a list of questions. She, of course, responded 'no' to all of them because she didn't know what he was talking about. Note that these were standard health history questions, like 'Did your mother have cancer?' How can they get an accurate health history if the patient to whom they are addressing the questions has memory loss?"

The Need for Compassion

Caregivers shared their views and pleas in an effort to help all professional caregivers and providers understand their feelings about having a loved one with Alzheimer's disease.

"I am presently a family caregiver who thinks doctors need to be available to just listen, or refer people to someone who will listen

to caregivers, as well as patients, especially when the diagnosis is first made," suggests a former nurse.

"My doctor has been great," comments a caregiver, *"but doctors need to understand it is not just our loved one with Alzheimer's disease who is confused. We family members are all grasping for help with understanding this disease."*

"My doctor's reaction to my concerns about my mother-in-law's memory loss and personality changes were met with very supportive answers to our questions. He spoke slowly and patiently with my mother-in-law," defends this caregiver. She continues with regret, *"Unfortunately, there just wasn't a whole lot of information available for us."*

A young granddaughter expresses her pain this way:

"Doctors could be a little less harsh and more gentle with some things they say. They need to know it would be so much more comforting to see them act kindly with my grandpa as well as with us. It's not that they are straight-out rude, but they should try to a little harder to make the extra effort because we are all hurting so much inside."

"Doctors, please try to understand that a person with Alzheimer's disease can still be loved," implores a caregiver, *"even though they are confused or have memory problems."*

Another family caregiver continues the pleas:

"Doctors need to understand persons with Alzheimer's disease have the right to use the rest of their lives being loved and cared for— and that is all right with us family members! But we need to know we have a physician's support."

This caregiver agrees:

"Physicians need to know Alzheimer's patients deserve quality of life. They are able to communicate some needs and wants even in the later states. BELIEVE IN THEM - - show them you care. They need that from you—and so do we."

☦

"Doctors need to know that family members do not want the person afflicted with Alzheimer's disease to simply be medicated and 'put away'," advises one special care unit volunteer. *"Families want to be kept abreast of what is happening and what to expect as each step progresses. Doctors seem unable or unwilling to do this."*

A nursing home administrator expresses her frustrations this way:

"One of the hardest things in caring for Alzheimer's patients in a nursing home is trying to understand why it takes so long for a doctor to get back to us on urgent matters. I sometimes think they consider our Alzheimer's residents less important just because they won't remember the delay in care. We caregivers know, and we really resent their lack of caring."

In support of that same concern, a caring nurse has this to add:

"Making nurses, families, and patients wait two to three days before they return phone calls on a resident who has Alzheimer's disease, causes everyone a lot of heartache. Why can't doctors realize that people with Alzheimer's disease who reside in nursing homes are important too, and deserve decent, attentive care."

An interesting comparison by another caregiver/daughter revealed:

"I found nursing home staff are more equipped than doctors to counsel and understand this disease. The first doctor I went to said 'Well, I can't do a thing for him (my dad).' The second doctor was more helpful. Then the nursing home staff led me to a compassionate understanding of my Dad's needs and care."

This caregiver shares her insight with:

"I wish doctors would understand the most important thing to a caregiver is the BEST care for their loved one. It may not be very important to the physician, but to the caregiver, it is the ONLY concern. I cannot just accept a physician saying to me, 'It just doesn't matter any more.' IT DOES MATTER!!!"

In support of her family physician who does understand, this caregiver tells a hopeful story:

"When I asked my physician for more medications to calm my aggressive father-in-law, he asked me if the drugs were for me, or the patient. He stopped me in my tracks when I heard him ask the staff to assist me in contacting support groups for my own therapy. I was so happy to see how much he really cared—about me!"

Hospitalization Problems

A number of surveys reflected the concerns of caregivers about the lack of knowledge on the part of professional hospital staff caring for a person who has Alzheimer's disease:

"I have just experienced the worst situations with my 90-year-old Mom who has Alzheimer's disease," one daughter relates. *"She had pneumonia and had to spend 10 days in the hospital. The problem? The hospital staff do not know how to care for a person who has Alzheimer's disease! They do not understand this awful disease and therefore lack adequate caring and coping skills. They need to be educated! We found that as a family, we needed to be there with Mom around the clock, to speak up for her and be her voice in this otherwise chaotic attempt to assist her. Mom didn't understand what was happening. And the staff didn't understand how to react to her."*

"Most hospital staff have never received adequate training in the care of a person with Alzheimer's disease," defends one nurse. *"This can be devastating for Alzheimer's persons who needs to be hospitalized. Alzheimer's disease is not the primary diagnosis during most hospitalizations, however the needs for understanding the patient with Alzheimer's disease are vital. Certainly a doctor or nurse would not ignore the 'Diabetes' secondary diagnosis on a chart. So it is that 'Alzheimer's disease' needs the prior acknowledgment and continuity of care."*

"In most hospitals, it is this elderly population who are coming in for hip and knee surgeries and replacements, pneumonia, and other acute medical problems," a family member points out. *"With 50 percent of those over 85 with Alzheimer's disease, we cannot emphasize the need for staff education and training enough. It is up to us to use our examples of prior hospitalizations of our loved ones to emphasize and alert the administrations to our needs."*

Caregiver Suggestions to Physicians

Several caregivers expressed their opinions by offering suggestions to improve the patient-doctor-family relationship and promote understanding. The following insightful remark comes from a family caregiver who had observed the care of her father over several years:

"I wish doctors, nurses and social workers better understood that these (people with Alzheimer's) are still human beings with feelings and emotions. Health professionals who work with this population should be mandated to receive continuing education and possibly periodic sensitivity training to learn how to approach and kindly manage those with dementia and their families. They should also strive to become much better listeners and seek out family members who are more familiar with the individuals' physical, emotional, and social history in order to determine the best treatment approach. In addition, physicians and nurses should not be so quick to utilize major medications as a control measure before trying behavioral management approaches."

A familiar problem vented by families is presented in this suggestion:

"Physicians need to know how to talk to patients and caregivers, patiently and repeatedly. Often they treated my mother-in-law clinically, but since Alzheimer's disease is a mental problem, they didn't want to approach the subject. They just need to be more supportive."

A granddaughter requests this of doctors who rely solely on standardized verbal memory testing:

"Take time to explain <u>everything</u>, not just to the patient, but to the family. Do not assume the standard verbal testing is adequate for all individuals. In my case, my Grandfather had been given the standard questions concerning recent events. These questions have been BS!!! He has never had an interest in sports, politics and other so-called 'normal' events which occur around him. He has always followed other things in life. But the doctors seem to think that this is abnormal. I am not making this up. We have been told that his lack of interest/knowledge indicates that he is extremely advanced in his Alzheimer's disease. Just because someone has no idea who won the World Series, who is playing in the Super Bowl, or who the current President might be, is not necessarily disconnected from reality."

Another caregiver suggests this remedy:

"Remember, the family (if close-knit) often will have the BEST idea of what the patient's interests and hobbies are. Use their knowledge to tailor your questions to EACH PATIENT!!!!!"

A care provider in a nursing home shares this remark:

"Doctors need to know that when their patient is being seen by another doctor, the doctors need to communicate with each other so they can make sure that all the medications that are being given are not going to hurt their patient. They also need to take time to listen, <u>really</u> listen, to their patients and to us caregivers when we talk, because we know our patients and their situations best of all. We are always seeking helpful ways to communicate our patients' needs to each doctor."

"Doctors need to know they have to treat the whole disease not just the medical conditions," admonishes another family member. *"Our neurologist thinks that his only job is to prescribe medication. He is reclusive and unhelpful in all other areas. This is very important.*

❧

We are looking for answers, not medication 'Band-Aids'."

"*Doctors need to understand the family is the most important link to their patient with Alzheimer's disease,*" states one daughter. "*My mother moved four years ago after my dad died suddenly and without warning. We saw the changes right after her move, although Mom was in denial. It took a year to convince her doctor Mom needed anti-depression medication. He finally said he didn't realize she was depressed! He didn't know her and he didn't ask us, her children. Since she is on the medications, she is a little better; at least able to make it through the day without crying. That is a victory! The illness needs to be accepted as an illness not as a 'custodial problem'."*

This frustrated family member apparently encountered the following situations more than once:

"*My family hates it when doctors do these two things: discuss matters in front of my mom as if she was not in the same room, and tell us things that give us false hope. We've had physicians talk about my mother when she was right there to hear him say, 'She will do this...' or 'If this happens with her...' We know my mother won't always catch on, but she feels humiliated and even more frustrated when doctors don't address information or questions to HER. Also, doctors need to be HONEST. It didn't do our family any good to be told, 'Well, she should be all right for a few months. You probably won't notice any change.' Wrong! Within two months of diagnosis my mother could no longer drive, work, write checks or cook supper.*"

A nurse/daughter/caregiver for her mother writes:

"*Physicians need to understand that while the treatment of acute illness is essential, his/her focus must remain on the bio-psyco-social aspects of the patient. Maintaining the patient's independence while treating an acute problem is essential in not causing more losses for the patient.*"

"*I wish my doctors understood the advice they give us applies to them too. Talk TO the patient as you would talk to the caregiver.*"

Speak slowly to him, and give him the respect worthy of an adult," advises this caregiver. "

Perhaps the following caregiver found the answer for the frustrating lack of proper care:

"Most professionals want to treat Alzheimer's disease as a medical illness. They need to remember a person with Alzheimer's disease has lost brain functioning and will not be able respond to their attempts of medical treatment to take care of the problem."

Frustrations with the lack of funding for Alzheimer's disease care prompted this suggestion from a family caregiver:

"The Alzheimer's Association in this country pours most of its money into medical research which misses the complete point. The associations should look at the people who have the disease and the people who care for them. How about half of their money going to lobby for federal health money to help care for persons with Alzheimer's disease and to help educate physicians about their care."

Another caregiver speaks out with this insight in behalf of persons with Alzheimer's disease:

"People with Alzheimer's disease have a right to be angry or depressed if they are, and they do not need to be 'drugged' out of it. In my experience with my Mom, the typical drugs given to Alzheimer's patients cause <u>more</u> confusion and impairment. Doctors should stop trying to appease family members by giving more pills or doing more brain scans or EEG's. Those tests don't make any difference in care. More compassionate understanding from physicians would."

"Doctors need to understand that caregivers, as well as the victims of Alzheimer's disease, require care and support," says this caregiver, once again supporting the belief that the family needs just as much "care" as the patient.

On a more ethereal level, this caregiver suggests another approach:

"Perhaps someone will understand that Alzheimer's disease is a lot like other diseases of the spirit body requiring a life shift spiritual

approach. Do we have any physicians who might embrace this approach?"

"I wish doctors understood the person with dementia he is treating is not just a patient," this caregiver/daughter tries to explain about her dad. *"He belongs to a family who loves him and is looking out for his best interest. The families need to know that their doctor understands there is a* <u>person</u> *inside that patient's body; the only difference is the patient/person has a demented brain."*

One granddaughter writes:

"I think family history and psychosocial issues must be taken into account when a family is given an Alzheimer's disease diagnosis. Doctors need to know this is an issue which affects the entire family. The doctor should make the appropriate referrals to support groups or resource centers, not just assume families know where to turn."

Family caregivers desire to be informed or at least know where to go for information:

"I wish doctors had the resourcefulness to inform family members and caregivers about support groups, books, and other resources available to help them with the coping of the disease I call 'hell on earth.'"

For handling inadequately prepared hospital staff, one consultant urges family caregivers to do some prior planning before their loved one with Alzheimer's disease is admitted to the hospital. She says:

"Not only nurses, but all department staff need to know how to care for your loved one with Alzheimer's disease. From the x-ray technicians, to security, to volunteers, it is important for everyone to know how to handle Alzheimer's clients. WE know you cannot 'reason' with someone who has Alzheimer's disease. We also know that it is not up to you, the family caregiver to 1.) be in attendance 24 hours a day; or 2.) educate the staff. So I urge you to encourage staff education

and training by appealing to your local Alzheimer's Associations, or going directly to the hospital administrations with your requests and concerns."

Conclusion

The majority of persons with Alzheimer's disease are cared for by a family member who has been initiated into this role through "baptism by fire," so to speak. They have had to push for a diagnosis, search for truths and education, overcome obstacles of care and understanding, and fight for the rights of their loved ones with Alzheimer's disease.

These surveys reveal some very important considerations for health care professionals: the need to become better educated about Alzheimer's disease and the need to listen with compassion to patients and their families. The comments of care and concern here are written to bring about an understanding of what caregivers need from physicians. They need compassionate, educated professionals who will listen to their concerns, trust their observations, provide educated answers and supportive referrals and follow-ups. They need to be heard, understood, and supported by physicians who understand.

7
ADULT CHILDREN CAREGIVERS SPEAK OUT

When adult children take on the responsibility of caring for a parent who has Alzheimer's disease, all the rules seem to change. It certainly is a role-reversal, and feelings can range from euphoria for the opportunity to help, to extreme anger and resentment for having to be in the care position without a choice.

Caregiving for a parent is not a "job" one can complete in a given time, and then go on to something else. As the disease progresses, the parent needs more and more attention and supervision until it becomes a 24-hour a day job. One of the biggest dangers to adult children caregivers is falling ill due to stress because they have no time to themselves when caring for an adult with Alzheimer's disease. This disease may rob that once-coherent, intelligent parent of any understanding of familiar places and persons. This may result in the parent wandering about aimlessly, getting out of locked doors at night, getting lost in the neighborhood, yet communicating in such a way as to make others think he is perfectly coherent. It then seems to be a "caregiver problem" and not the person with a disease who needs help.

Many adult children are personally caring for their aging parents. They care for their parents in their own homes, in the parent's home, or in care facilities. With the alarming number of parents today who have Alzheimer's disease, the emotional, physical and financial strains are evident in the words of these caregivers. Many took the time and had the courage to share what their lives are really like. Keeping in mind the statistics from the Alzheimer's Association that says an estimated 50 percent of people who reach the age of 85 will have Alzheimer's disease, it is apparent to see why so many adult children are becoming responsible for their parents.

Many of these adult children are young parents themselves, with young families to support. These families "speak out" in the following chapters. More often, the adult children are retired and had anticipated some leisure time with their grown children, but instead they are faced with the decisions of direct care of their elderly parents with Alzheimer's disease.

Statistics show the person most likely to be the primary family caregiver for an aging parent is the eldest daughter or the wife of the eldest son. The National Center for Health Services statistical studies revealed about 70 percent of parents between the ages of 65 and 84 live near at least one of their children. After the age of 85, that number increases to 78 percent.

The frustration expressed most often by adult children of parents with Alzheimer's disease is they are "parenting their parent." In addition, many of these adult children not only have children, but also grandchildren, of their own for whom to care. They often feel "sandwiched in" as caregivers.

Compounding the emotions of adult-child caregiving are thoughts of the past parent-adult/child relationship through the years which has a major impact on the present relationship. If the struggles of the past were intense, the conflicts of the present issues are magnified when a parent is now in need of care.

It is important to understand that all parent-child relationships bear the hardship of stress at times. However, when a parent has Alzheimer's disease, the relationship forces parent-child reversal roles as the caregiver learns the adult being "parented" is indeed not a child. The elder parents come into this disease with all their many years of wisdom and experience, albeit lost or misinterpreted through the cruelty of the disease. As the disease progresses, and they require more care, the parents may sometimes act like children. The fact remains they are the parent and therefore always require one's respect and love. The heartfelt feelings and thoughts expressed here by adult children caregivers reflect the irony and conflict of this adult child-parent relationship.

Pleas for understanding

Adult children taking care of their parents represent an ever-growing segment of today's society. Many suffer in silence. Most plea for understanding from a society which often turns a deaf ear and lacks understanding.

"I wish everyone understood Alzheimer's disease is the most insidious, inconceivably destructive disease to both patient and caregivers," laments one despairing family caregiver. *"Its invisibility is not at all understood like illnesses that leave scars, or can be seen in a microscope. I just wish people could understand what years of gradual grieving do to a person who is losing the only other person in the world who has given unconditional love. The stress of caring for this person has meant slipping in and out of depression. How do I explain that to all of you? How can I get you to understand how I feel? I can't. So I carry on almost silently with a periodic urge to climb a hill and shout to everyone about how I feel. But I can't. You wouldn't understand anyway. How could you, when I don't understand it myself? I just wish everyone would understand . . . about Alzheimer's disease!"*

"My father and family need to understand the stress of caring for Mom has meant my lapsing in and out of depression," defends another daughter. *"'Focus on something else,' you say; 'Take care of yourself,' you say; 'Your Mom isn't the same person any more—she wouldn't want you to feel this way! I wish my family would try to understand. They just don't get it."*

Another daughter remarks:

"I wish society understood dealing with a family member with Alzheimer's disease is much more than dealing with a person who

has memory loss. It changes everything about the person. It also changes all of our lives more than other people could ever imagine."

One loving daughter-in-law has this to say:

"I wish our relatives understood that Mom is not doing this deliberately. She is not just being difficult. She can't help it. Yes, she repeats and repeats, yes she argues, yes she denies and yes it is terrible to deal with, but she's not doing this to make our lives miserable. Because I am an in-law and don't have a long history with my mother-in-law, I think I can deal better with this, although it is frustrating. What is doubly hard is dealing with my husband who takes her condition personally, and relatives who only know how to criticize.".

"We all need to realize how frightening and depressing it is for our parent with Alzheimer's disease," comments a family caregiver. *"How terrifying it must be to wake up and not know where you are or why you are there. Why can't my family realize this terror and understand my compassion instead of criticizing my care."*

Another adult daughter implores for understanding from her friends about her need to be a *person*, not always a caregiver:

"This is a demanding disease. I am bone tired. So is everyone else I know who is caregiving. Please don't ask me every time we meet, 'How is your mother?' You are for the most part, bored with the answer, even if I just say, 'About the same.' I am still a person; speak to ME. I have developed a zillion at-home hobbies and interests. Find out what they are and ask me about one of them. Ask me anything, but 'how is your mother?' I do not need to talk about her during every precious minute of freedom I have. I would like to leave thoughts of her 'at home' so I could feel like somebody in my own right, if only for those precious few hours a week when I am running my errands—without her."

The following two family caregivers plead for understanding from co-workers as they describe their lives as caregivers who also hold outside jobs:

❡

"I wish my co-workers would understand Alzheimer's disease is arguably more debilitating and frustrating for the caregiver than it is for the patient. It is the MOST stressful event I have ever encountered in my life. Words to describe the caregiving experience fail me. Caregiving consumes my entire life. The responsibilities and stress never leave me, even if I am physically removed from the situation. This stress cannot be put aside for a time. It is there every minute of my '36-hour day.'" (She is referring to Dr. Peter Rabins' book about caregiving, entitled "The 36-Hour Day.")

"My co-workers need to understand if I must take a leave of absence to try to gain some control of my life, please do not ostracize me. You do not know what I am experiencing because you have not had the same experience. How dare you judge me! I am doing what I think is right, what I think is best for my mother."

A fatigued-sounding family caregiver shares this thought:

"I wish others understood that the primary caregiver needs relief from time to time and that encouragement, no matter how small, is very necessary."

"Unless you are SUPER human, with unlimited strength and endurance, there is no possible way you alone can do all that needs to be done to care for a person with severe Alzheimer's disease," emphatically comments another caregiver. *"We all need help!"*

"I wish others would understood it is really harder for the families to handle this disease than it is for the person who has it," clarifies a family member.

"It's very hard for those close to mother, but not with her on a 24-hour basis, to understand her constantly changing requirements and needs," adds another caregiver.

"I wish my husband understood that many days I need to just get away," implores one daughter-in-law/caregiver. *"My mother-in-law has been living with us for over two years and prior to that I took care*

of her in an Alzheimer's wing of a local rest home. It is a very difficult job, with very little rewards."

Anger

Many adult children caregivers expressed their anger at their deplorable life situation and at the ignorance of those who don't take the time to understand.

"I can't take anymore! I have cared for my dad, and now my mom. Both have/had Alzheimer's disease. When do I get a life of my own and rest at night?" questions a weary daughter.

"It hurts so much to see my dad deteriorate. I look into his eyes and see . . . nothing. He is a hollow shell of a man. I am losing the memory of the person he used to be. This hurts so much. I know I'll never see him truly happy again. The anger and pain I feel runs so deeply," utters a grieving daughter. *"I feel gypped. Where is the nurturing, happy father and grandfather we all so desperately need now? I am angry for us and for him!"*

"My aunt just sent a 'get well' card to my mom, her sister, who is in a special care nursing home for those with Alzheimer's disease. It made me so angry! Don't they understand that Mom is not SICK. Are they living in the dark ages? Mom is strong and healthy, but has a brain disease from which she will never recover. 'Get well' seems so inappropriate!" a daughter submits.

"I am seething with anger! Some nice 'caring souls' at the Senior Citizens Center who believed every word my mother with dementia fabricated and told them, turned me into Social Services for abuse! You got it! I was sitting here at my computer, minding my own business, when the case worker rang the door bell. I was investigated for abuse. As if that wasn't enough, about eight months later someone else turned me in again. I know these' nice' senior citizens really believed my mother's stories of abuse, but I would never

hurt my mom. I offered to let them live with her for about a month, so they could see what it is really like with her fabricating stories. There were NO TAKERS!"

One distraught daughter, who was also a physician, expressed her anger this way:

"The worst part was not knowing how quickly the disease was going to progress. Also, not knowing when it would take Dad's life. I wish I had known how much he had to suffer with the disease. It was like he had died three years ago, at the onset of this disease. I hated how he couldn't recognize everyone and I hated that I could not do anything to help him."

"I wish someone would have told me earlier that my mother had Alzheimer's disease," laments another daughter. *"When I went to see her (2200 miles away) I just found out she probably has had Alzheimer's disease for years! I am very angry at the doctor. When she went into the nursing home a few months later, she was also diagnosed with lung and colon cancer. Why didn't the doctor tell us! It is very frustrating!"*

"I have a family who is in total denial about mom's Alzheimer's disease," this daughter relates. *"I get so angry when they don't even call me to give me moral support. I have come to realize that each caregiver has to handle things in his/her own way. My son hates to visit because he doesn't want to see Mom the way she is now; the far-off relatives don't see where there's much of a problem because Mom is not yet in a hospital or nursing home. Strangers don't even think there is anything wrong with mother! But luckily for me, my husband is wonderfully understanding."*

Feelings of Guilt

Feelings of guilt on the part of caregivers, especially adult-children caregivers, are often hidden, ignored, or denied: *"I must not be doing enough!" or "I don't know how to do it right." "I even question my love for this person, because she has interfered with my life." "I do love this person, but I struggle with the thoughts of wanting him to die."*

Guilt. Guilt about the care they are giving. Guilt about the ugly thoughts that life would be easier without that parent. Guilt about the need to engage the help of others outside the family. It touches the soul when we come to realize these good, giving family members are antagonizing over deep feelings of guilt.

"My guilt is the feelings of anger I have as I realize I am missing out on many pleasures of life. I am feeling resentful. I have even blamed my husband for doing this to me (my having to care for his mother in our home). That is so unfair to him because he is so kind and loving to me. Then I feel resentment toward his mother because I am losing special times with my girls. I am tired, depressed, and ill-tempered and it ruins our time together. We used to be so close, my mother-in-law and I. Now I resent her intruding into our lives. We once had a happy home. I hate the idea of putting her in a home and everyone else in the family does too, and she won't want to either. I really don't know how to handle these guilty feelings of mine!"

"I am feeling totally swallowed up by my own situation with my 88-year-old mother-in-law. She is not regressing rapidly as so many others her age are. I feel I am consumed with depression, frustration and guilt!!! I feel I can no longer cope. I want to scream or cry."

Often times the admittance of guilt and the resolve of its blame does not occur until after a parent's death:

"I hesitate to share this thought, but the truth is, I felt an immense sense of relief after my father finally died."

"I could never have <u>caused</u> my father's death. However, I do not grieve with guilty feelings over my decision to prevent procedures that would have delayed his death and suffering."

🎗

Caregivers often share this feeling, along with their feeling of shame or guilt for wishing their parent's death. It is good to open up to those feelings and find a safe haven to express such feelings. It is understandable to want your parent out of misery. It is equally understandable to think about seeking peace for yourself. Support groups around the world offer caregivers who will understand your feelings, hold your hand and tell you it's OK to have those feelings. They will further validate such feelings by telling you that they too endured such feelings as caregivers for their parents.

Two experienced caregivers, acknowledging their guilt, offer words of comfort and support to adult-children caregivers:

"If you ever had children, you can recall the sleepless nights, walking a crying baby, fighting to stay awake, and experiencing feelings of love and resentment at the same time. Did that make you a bad parent? Of course not. So I find comfort in knowing that, even though I detest my Mother's illness, and the fact that she keeps me up nights with her wandering and questions, my feelings of resentment are just that—FEELINGS. And that's OK."

"I think guilt is a constant companion to those of us with loved ones with Alzheimer's disease. But we all DO have lives of our own and other family members who need us. So we do the best we can and we continue to offer all the support and love we can to our elderly parents. If we can find satisfaction in knowing we are doing the best we can, that is all we can hope for at this time."

Conflicts

It often is the very absurdity of life's new situations which cause mental conflict about an adult child's new role as parent-caregiver. Caregivers express their feeling of conflict in the many decisions they are left to make on behalf of their parents with Alzheimer's disease. Conflict arises, not only in the decision process, but with the disapproval of others once the decision is made.

"I wish everyone would understand family takes care of family, and NO, I can't just put my Mother 'away' and forget her!" a defiant caregiver explains.

"I don't know how to handle my Dad who has Alzheimer's disease. His schedule doesn't conform to our family's schedule. The activities, number of people, noise and surroundings in our normal home seems to worsen his condition by increasing stress as the disease progresses. I'm at a loss as to where to turn."

"I would like to know what kind of an establishment you are to put your parent into when she is in the beginning stages of Alzheimer's? My Mom currently lives at home alone with help throughout the day. Knowing Mom is going to have to be 'put away' because she also has other problems with her health, I have done my investigation of local facilities. Yet I still do not kmow which way to go, and knowing that the time is growing very near, I fear I'll make the wrong decision," a concerned son shares about his conflicts.

"The hardest thing for me," states a devastated son, *"was having to take my Dad's keys away. He loved his cars and had been a good driver for many years. It was a very emotional moment when he handed over his keys to me. It's not a thing I ever thought I would have to demand of him. It was like his final act of independence—and now he is totally dependent. It hurts me so much as it still causes conflict between us."*

"Chances are I will never be satisfied with the decisions I have made in the care of my mother," another adult child comments. *"I will always wonder if I could have done something better or different. With Alzheimer's disease, we never know if these are the BEST decisions, because there are none. No decision will really make a difference, for the end is always the same."*

"I am doing the best I can. Feeling guilty will not help me. I have to find a balance between mom's needs and mine. I can't control

or stop this disease, so there are limits to how much I can help," justifies this caregiver facing conflict.

"Anyone who cares for an Alzheimer's victim 24 hours a day deserves a medal," comments another caregiver. She goes on to describe her life of discord, *"People not close to me don't realize how hard it is to keep my sanity. Fortunately, we need to spend only four to five hours a day with Mom at this time. However, when it becomes necessary to give more time to her, I'm afraid we will have to look to nursing home care because I will never be able to cope."*

Mental anxiety and conflict are apparent in this caregiver's interpretation:

"The hardest part for me in dealing with this terrible disease is watching my Mom not being able to do certain things that she had always done. Even worse than that is watching her try to 'cover up' for her inabilities. What do I do? I play her game and act like I don't even notice her disabilities. Somehow it makes me feel like I'm helping Mom this way. Is it wrong?"

"Nothing prepares you for the awful effects Alzheimer's has on your own life, as well as on the person who is affected. It is one crisis after another that needs resolve and decisions," an exhausted caregiver voices.

"My father-in-law and I once shared a commonality of the medical profession. Today it is so difficult to see someone who was once a health professional and a colleague lose his mental acuity. I wasn't prepared for the devastating effect Alzheimer's disease has on my father-in-law. He knows something is wrong, but he can't figure out what has gone wrong. Everything has become difficult for him, and he becomes very depressed over little things. This is what's so hard for me to handle," admits a loving daughter-in-law.

"The societal stigma and discrimination was something I was not prepared for," another family caregiver confesses.

Daily episodes cause discord that adds to the conflicts of normal care. One of the problems is forgetfulness which leads to hiding things in unlikely places:

"Right now we are going into our winter, and they are even forecasting sleet and possibly snow tonight. Once again my Mother has hidden her winter coat. I have already looked in all the obvious places, so next I guess I turn the house upside down trying to find it for her. It would be nice if I could just afford to go buy her a new one. Since we are on a very limited fixed income, I can't possibly replace everything that she 'loses'. Of course, she says she didn't touch it, so she doesn't have any idea what happened to it."

"I had to restrain myself from becoming angry when she kept forgetting where she left her rings, or information about an event that was to take place within a short time frame."

Another source of conflict is the constant repetition by the person with Alzheimer's:

"The worst part is having to repeat an answer to the same question that has been asked a hundred times, without sounding frustrated. Added to that is the conflict I feel within when I have to take the false criticism from my mom without striking back in defense of myself."

"I wish someone would have told me earlier the phases in which an Alzheimer's patient goes through and what to expect as the disease progresses. I feel in constant conflict trying to 'outguess' this disease," a frustrated caregiver admits.

Another caregiver describes conflict with personal emotions:

"The saddest times were when my mother would forget loved ones that had passed on and kept asking where they were. Part of me wanted to scream out with 'How could you forget they died! The other part of me fought such conflicting feelings, and patiently reminded her of some happy event with that person."

"Be strong, yet don't be afraid to cry," encourages an adult caregiver. *"I believe conflicting feelings are all a part of caregiving. My advice: educate, educate, educate yourself about this disease! Then share your knowledge with others."*

Fears and Worries

Adult children have may fears and worries before, during, and after the diagnosis of Alzheimer's disease. Several took the time to share their anxieties about getting Alzheimer's disease themselves. Others feared for the safety of their loved ones with Alzheimer's disease, and family who lived with them.

"Not all Alzheimer's disease is inherited. My sister and I have spent too many hours worrying about our own minor memory lapses before we learned the facts," one daughter relates.

"When I first heard the diagnosis, I kept asking myself: Is it curable? Is it contagious? Can it be passed down through the genes and on whose side? Why does my husband's family have so many relatives with Alzheimer's disease on his mother's side of the family?" questions one wife.

"When I first got my Dad's diagnosis of Alzheimer's disease I thought 'Oh no!' I was very scared and I had a right to be. This disease is a very scary thing!" justifies a son/caregiver.

"When Mum first got her diagnosis, I had already worked professionally with the disease for the previous six years. I was devastated! Fear and panic over the future gripped me, and the lonely journey began and has not yet ended," laments a frightened daughter.

"It was so devastating to find out Mom's diagnosis," explains another daughter. *"Not only do you learn that you will never recover the health of your loved one, you also have to make a load of decisions about your own life, and your parent's life. All this, while fearing you might be the next one to get Alzheimer's disease."*

"My mother lived with us for nine months, wandering out of our home several times a day. That was tolerable, although very time-consuming," this daughter remarks. *"Then she started to get mean. When we became afraid she would hurt the grandchildren, we placed her in a nursing home. That was one of the hardest decisions I ever had to make in my life!"*

Fears about making the right choices regarding the living arrangements for a parent with Alzheimer's disease are very apparent in these comments:

"When I first heard the words 'Alzheimer's disease' my thoughts were: she is going to die!" a terrified daughter recalls. *"That was three years ago and she is still on her own. I'm scared to death she will hurt herself or make a mistake in her medications, but she keeps going on. I'm thankful for that. It's giving me the time I need to educate myself and to get my siblings out of denial!"*

"I just don't know if we are committing a grave or dangerous error by permitting my mother-in-law to stay alone in her apartment, even if we phone and visit daily. She loses things constantly and then tells us 'a ghost took them.' She calls me in the evening and totally forgets we had spent the day together. She even forgets I am married to her son! Yet most of the time, we have very meaningful conversations and I feel very close to her. I worry constantly about her safety alone. My husband believes if we ever put her in a nursing home, she will just die. I just cannot seem to ascertain what a responsible level of promoting independence and caring for her at the same time should be."

Sometimes the fears become realities when the behavior shows signs of danger:

"The last time I left Mother alone was to go to an Alzheimer's seminar, and when I came home she had shampooed her hair. She had the stove burner turned on, and when I asked her what she was

doing, she replied, 'I'm drying my hair.'   If I had not come home when I did, I shutter to think what could have happened!"

Financial/Legal Concerns

Some family caregivers shared comments about the necessity to learn and understand financial and legal situations affecting their parent with Alzheimer's disease:

"I wish someone would have told me earlier that I may have to care for my parents in a financial way," this caregiver laments. *"I am a nurse, yet I had no idea of the financial burden Alzheimer's disease could cause in a family until it happened to us."*

"My mother-in-law can't afford the medication my father-in-law, who has Alzheimer's disease, is presently taking. We three children take turns buying the medication. My father-in-law doesn't realize this. My mother-in-law will not tell us children when the medication is out, because she is embarrassed with their financial situation. She has refused to read any literature or attend any lectures or support groups to learn more about Alzheimer's disease. Instead, she calls her son, my husband, with complaints about having to make all the decisions in the house, and her husband won't help her. We can't make her understand that he can no longer make such decisions, not that he doesn't want to!"

"The most frustrating thing about Alzheimer's disease is there is no legal protection for us," a caregiver learns. *"My mother paid every bill that came in on the same day it arrived and unfortunately it included all junk mail like sweepstakes, awards, contests, solicitation, and fund raisers! She ended up spending $750 (as of last April) monthly on junk mail! To make a long story short, I ended up filing a petition for guardianship; the judge looked at her, asked her few questions, then turned down my petition. The court-appointed lawyer said it was her right to pay for sweepstakes, awards, contests,*

etc. as much as it was the right of people who want to spend money on the lottery. I was unable to get any legal action to protect my mother in her incompetence. It was financially devastating to us."

Common Frustrations

Adult children share about the frustrations of daily events:

"My husband says I should overlook the small things. I know I should but it is the small things that throw me for a loop. Small things like my mother-in-law breaking my good dishes when she tries to 'help' me in the kitchen; opening a second container of milk before the first one is finished; piling clothes in her closet floor so that the door will not even close; not closing the shower curtain so that water is everywhere when she finishes. I know this sounds trivial, but the list goes on and on, and I don't know how to handle these things. I don't know how to ignore all this!" a wife tries to explain.

Several caregivers relayed frustration caused by living and working in a distant city separating them from their parent with Alzheimer's disease:

"I can no longer talk to the father I knew. He has no words. My mother, who is the direct caregiver, is overwhelmed and depressed by his situation. I feel powerless, as I am 3,000 miles from home and can go there only once a year."

"The most frustrating thing is being unable to help because I live and work so far away. When I called my Mom, she would claim my father had kidnapped her to an unknown place, which in reality was the home they had lived in for more than seven years! It tore me up to hear her accusations while I try to counsel and support my Dad across the phone lines."

"The most frustrating part is living 2,200 miles away from my mother who has Alzheimer's disease. I feel powerless to assist in her care, but I cannot move or change jobs at this time."

Not only distance separates family from their loved ones with Alzheimer's disease. One family caregiver expresses it this way:

"It is mostly memory which links us all together as family or friends. Even though I live in the same city as my Mom, the separation of people because of the destruction of memory just tears me apart."

Caregivers went on to share common frustrations as adult children trying to meet the needs of their parents:

"One of the most disturbing things about Alzheimer's disease is that you are never sure your parent really has it, until it is too late," a caregiver notes.

"The most frustrating thing for me is meeting the special needs of my mother as a deaf person who has Alzheimer's disease," this daughter shares. *"I am deaf myself. Mother's family doctor demanded I get an interpreter, but when I get one, he refused to pay, saying the cost was too high. I took her to a different doctor, a Geriatrician this time, and he was very good about meeting our needs with interpreters. The social worker also arranged to have home care visits by a nurse with an interpreter since there are no relatives around. They (the doctor and social worker) strongly recommended I place Mom either in an assisted living facility or nursing home where there is a program for the deaf. There is only one in the U.S. to my knowledge. That one has a five-year waiting list. I know of two other places which admit deaf people and have some staff who can communicate in sign language. One is in a hometown about ten miles from where my mother lives. They could not admit her against her will and said I needed guardianship before I can admit her. The court denied it so I had no place to go. I feel like I always get the royal run-around. Nothing is easy!"*

"One of the saddest things that happened was when my Mom could not remember she had just asked for my help," a daughter recalls. *"She cannot seem to remember anything that happens within a 20-minute time span. At times she starts abusing me verbally as though it is I who does not know what reality is. This is so frustrating because there is no good way to handle this."*

"Alzheimer's disease makes the person afflicted suspicious, angry, paranoid and depressed. Usually the people who care for them (like myself) are the ones who are targets of these emotions. We don't deserve it, but what are we to do?" another daughter asks.

"We adult children need to have some information about how the disease will affect our loved ones so they can make the most of their lucid moments," this caregiver notes. *"But trying to get good information is very time-consuming and frustrating."*

"The most frustrating thing is my mother-in-law's unwillingness to accept this disease my father-in-law has," remarks another family member. *"She feels like we shouldn't talk about it, or even recognize it's existence. She refuses to read any literature on the disease process, then continually whines and complains to her children that her spouse is acting in a certain way that he has never acted before."*

"The most frustrating thing was seeing the negative personality changes in my dad, and trying to deal with them," a loving son relates.

"Talk about frustration! I was never mentally and physically prepared to understand that someone I've known all of my life, who has been strong and independent, will need to depend on me for everything and will not even remember I am his daughter," this caregiver cries.

Another caregivers vents her frustration in these words:

"Caregiving for another person is the most difficult of jobs. It is a 24-hour a day job, and it is not going to change until the loved one is taken away through death. It truly is a 'long good-bye.' I know through personal experience."

"Mom has no memory left at all," voices a heavy-hearted daughter. *"It is so sad. She still recognizes my sister and me, but rarely remembers our names."*

"My dad thinks it is just <u>one</u> thing he needs to change in his

life, and his troubles with memory loss will be over," another disappointed daughter explains. *" He thinks 'If I can just get rid of that housekeeper, I'll be cured. Or, if I could just start writing again, I'll be fine.' It's so frustrating for him —and for me."*

"He needs to quit driving. He needs to be nicer to Mom. He needs to quit waking Mom up! But he can't—and there is nothing we can do. How frustrating!" this family member sums up the discords in their lives.

The strife of everyday living takes on new meaning when living with a person who has Alzheimer's disease:

"I had Caller ID which was new. When I started getting calls from strangers asking me who had called from this number, I knew it was time to take away the phone. She proceeded to tell anyone who would listen to her that I locked her in her room and wouldn't let her make any phone calls. She also added that I was stealing all of her things. The latter was because I had gone through her clothing drawers and 'confiscated' three hammers, numerous screw drivers, pliers, nails, screws, a pocket knife, and miscellaneous other articles. By the way, did I mention that people with Alzheimer's disease like to 'pack rat' things away?"

"The saddest thing that happened was when my mother-in-law tried to pick up crafts that she used to do routinely and sat with everything in her lap and cried because she didn't know what to do or how to do it. When I tried to show her, she couldn't begin to do it. She cried more and begged me to put her away. It broke my heart," a daughter remarks.

"The most frustrating part is my mother-in-law's inability to retain information, her constant repetitive questions, and her denial of any wrong-doing," comments a family caregiver.

"Alzheimer's patients are very adept at acting quite normal when they are around strangers," cautions a caregiver with experience.

"My mother used to go to the Senior Citizens Center which gave me a few hours to run errands. They thought she was a delightful old lady. Little did they know I had just put a lock on the back door so she couldn't get out without me knowing because she would wander away, not being able to find her way back home."

Other adult children express their frustrations in these quotes:

"I wish someone would have told me earlier I would feel so ineffective, so helpless, so frustrated!"

"The worst part is having to deal with the crazy thinking or the combativeness all the time. It is extremely draining on both my mother and I."

"The most frustrating thing about Alzheimer's is the roller coaster of good days/ bad days. One day my mother will be coherent and go shopping and be laughing; the next day (or even later the same day) she will stare at the coffee pot not knowing where to pour the water, or worse yet, go into the closet instead of the bathroom."

"Alzheimer's is such a hard disease, not only on the person who has it, but on the caregiver. You watch the person become less and less able to care for herself and turn into someone you do not even know. My mother had to come live with us after living alone for thirty years. She didn't realize what was wrong with her. We brought her to Florida from New York. As the disease progressed she would walk out of my house at least ten times a day. She thought she was walking 'home' to New York which she believed was right around the corner. There were times I would get so frustrated, I would want to just let her keep walking. Each time I would get in my car, follow her until she was too tired to walk anymore, and then she would finally get into my car and come back home, only to rest up and leave again!"

"I wish my mother would understand I am doing everything humanly possible to provide a safe, secure, and pleasant environment for her to live within, and that I am trying my very best to comply with her wishes every step of the way."

🎗

"Nothing will work all the time with an Alzheimer's patient, just as nothing will consistently work with a spoiled two-year-old. I have often compared my mother to that. Sometimes I feel like I am going through the terrible two's with an adult."

From day-to-day events, to frustrations with abnormal adult behavior, family caregivers are stressed out. Read on for a better understanding of other specific frustrations facing adult children caregivers.

Frustrations With the Government

"I wish someone would have told me earlier that society and government bodies were so ignorant of the pain and suffering of those with a dementing illness," states a caregiver. *"They are equally as ignorant of the needs for support for caregivers and significant others."*

"I wish politicians could grasp the fact that if a caregiver is willing to keep the family member with Alzheimer's disease at home, it takes a toll on both patient and caregiver They shouldn't make it so hard to get a home attendant, even part time. Not all children with a parent suffering from this disease are willing to help care for their parent at home. The ones who help shouldn't be further punished. The current rules, especially in New York, are a disgrace!" a family caregiver points out.

"My mother was killed in a car wreck and now the only person I have left is my father. Unfortunately, he cannot remember anything. The most frustrating thing is that there are cures but government will not allow people to know about them. (I believe) mercury fillings and other metals cause Alzheimer's and the sooner the American Dental Association recognizes it, the better!" this caregiver says.

Some caregivers address the need for our nation to take notice of the four million people in the United States with Alzheimer's disease:

"Alzheimer's is a disease about which the nation and each individual needs to become concerned. With the aging of Americans, more people will become afflicted with this disease each year.

Resources need to be located to fund research, educate the public, provide respite care for caregivers, and establish suitable facilities for the care of Alzheimer's patients."

"Seeing what they (the government) spend on trivial things like space flights makes me ill. What good are rocks from the moon when we have four million citizens with Alzheimer's disease, and their families, in need their help right here?" another caregiver comments with disgust.

"I wish those who make the decisions about Medicare and Medicaid understood Alzheimer's disease is a DISEASE which destroys discretely functional neural activities. As renal failure is covered by Medicare, so should Alzheimer's disease be included in a similar aid program which could minimize the brutal destruction of what is left of my family," one caregiver offers as a suggestion.

"I wish the government would understand people with Alzheimer's disease deserve care with dignity and love," adds a compassionate adult-child caregiver. *"Our government succeeds in supporting entitlement programs for those who are ill and have their mental capacities, yet fails to protect those who are helpless because of their mental decline."*

"The only way we will make the progress we need is to work with the Alzheimer's Association. Only as one united voice are we strong," encourages one family caregiver.

Families who thought they could rely on government help through Medicare for their aging parents are discovering there is no aid for people who "just have Alzheimer's disease." This not only causes financial hardships, but stressful home relationships for the entire family.

Frustrations with Care Facilities

Sometimes, many times sadly enough, everything a caregiver does is not enough. Parents with Alzheimer's disease are no longer the same parents who told their children of their wishes prior to the disease onset.

⚑

As the disease progresses, no matter how safe, secure and pleasant the environment is, it may not be safe and secure enough to protect a parent with Alzheimer's disease from harm. The ugly nature of this disease causes a person to forget what had been decided upon at an earlier conversation or what was told to them just minutes ago.

The adult child must make decisions for a parent who is putting his or her life or health in jeopardy, just as real as when they were the young child of that parent who made decisions for them. No matter how much a parent with this disease protests or begs, if it is not in their best interest to care for them at home, one MUST step in and ignore previous declarations about going into a nursing care facility.

"It's a compromise," justifies this family caregiver. *"Sometimes the family has to give up the loving one-on-one care we were previously able to offer at home, and settle for the 'generic,' SAFER care provided at a nursing home, regardless of our parent's wishes."*

Placement in a nursing home facility, however, often does not bring the peace family caregivers expected:

"How I wish nursing home staffs were better trained! I've been the caregiver for my step-dad for five years. I became his caregiver after my mom was hospitalized. She was hospitalized for a whole year: three months in ICU and nine months in a sub-acute unit. I cared for him because he has Alzheimer's disease and because he required around-the-clock care at home and couldn't be left alone. I believe his wandering is what put my mom in the hospital in the first place, and eventually ended her life due to respiratory failure, then heart failure. Six months after her passing, I had to place my step-dad in a nursing home, after a short hospital stay. I had no choice of nursing homes because my dad was placed on Medi-cal. Instead of giving me the peace of mind I needed, the nursing home has been a nightmare for me!" They have no empathy for me as his family caregiver."

X

"Professional caregivers need to realize not all Alzheimer's patients are the same, just as not all cardiac patients are the same," advises a family member. *"With Alzheimer's disease, as with most dementia, the only way to truly discover the best care is by asking the patient. If the patient is confused and can't give you a straight answer, you have to use your skills of observation to understand the patient, or better yet, ask the family."*

"I'm only one person so I could not be there (at the care facility) every day. I have a family with a 10-year-old son who has A.D.H.D. and a husband who had a heart attack last July. Every time I went it seemed the staff would be yelling at my Dad as if he couldn't hear. I told them over and over that his hearing is fine; he has ALZHEIMER'S. Why don't THEY understand?!" another family member cries.

Family members were equally concerned with physicians' response time to meet the needs of their loved ones in a care facility:

"A family member expresses concern for a condition of a nursing home patients, then the nursing home calls the doctor. They leave a message with the answering service. The physician usually waits until the next day to answer this (non-emergency) message, and then he leaves orders for a prescription. Then the pharmacy is called and brings the prescription whenever they make their regular deliveries, which could be the next day. That means, for example, that a bladder infection could take 2-3 days before the medication is administered to the patient. The feeling among some caregivers and some nursing home staff personnel is that many doctors just are not very responsive. Not all patients have family members available to shortcut the system and help get the medication sooner."

"Once he fell out of bed in the care facility and had a very banged up arm," tells a concerned daughter. *"I asked them if the physician had given him anything for pain. Their answer was 'he had not complained of pain.' I told them, 'Of course he won't <u>complain</u> of pain; he can't even <u>ask</u> for a glass of water!"*

✗

"The saddest thing that happened was my mother fell and broke her wrist after only one and a half weeks in the nursing home. She is a very gifted pianist and had just started playing for the residents. She has been going downhill ever since, and cannot even get out of bed on her own any longer. She is expected to die in the next month. Could all of this have been prevented?!" questions a saddened family member.

Sometimes the answer is simple, and a comment to the physician can make all the difference:

"My dad lost five pounds in one month at the nursing home. I questioned this since whenever I came in to feed him, he had been eating 80-100 percent of his food. When the doctor talked to staff about his feeding, he gained two pounds the very next month. He has to have someone feed him and I feel they just weren't feeding him."

One family member requests this from her mother's caregivers:

"I want to be consulted when you change Mom's medications, move my mom to another room, are unable to have her hair done as scheduled, or send her to a hospital. I am no longer a daughter, I am my mother's mother. You would not do these things to my child without my permission. These situations are no different. My frustration with your refusal to do this is very real and very hard to live with. The best surprise is no surprises. I am in your facility twice a week. A note could be left with the desk. You could phone me at work. You could phone me at home. When I come to take my mom out to dinner, I would like to eat the meal without being angry or upset because you handed me 'surprises,'" vents a overwhelmed daughter.

Many caregivers in the facilities do not take the time to inform a son or daughter about the day-to-day changes of their parent. The frustrations adult children feel when leaving a loved one in the hands and care of a facility are very real. It is very much like leaving a child in the care of a sitter. A lack of communication can cause even more frustrations and hardships as demonstrated in this scenario:

"Last Friday I got a call from Dad's nursing home saying he had started coughing Thursday night and they called his doctor who told them to put him on antibiotics and oxygen. When I went to see him I was told that because of the pneumonia, he had had a heart attack. At the hospital they did blood work and it showed that there was an enzyme change which I know (from my husband's heart attack) takes at least 18 hours to show after the heart attack. The heart attack was brought on by low oxygen saturation in the blood, according to what his doctor told me. He is still struggling along. At 86 years old and in the late stages of Alzheimer's, I don't know how long he has. I talked to his doctor today and I told him I do not want him returning to the nursing home he was in! I will try and find another one and see if his doctor will sign an order for hospice. I tried this when we saw the weight drop, but his doctor wouldn't sign saying he wasn't terminal! I'm beside my self! I have no support! Even though my step-dad has four natural adult children, none of them have come to see him since all of this started five years ago . . . another story altogether." This is the type of script that is common to the frustrations of adult children caregivers as they struggle with decisions regarding the everyday care of their parent.

"There is a need for a type of care facility which is beyond the independence of assisted living, yet not as structured or confined as a nursing home," a family member proposes. Chapter 15 in this book will help define the various types of facilities, giving caregivers added information for their educated decisions regarding the care of their loved ones.

The decision about placement is never easy, and once made, a whole new litany of frustrations may begin:

"I felt so inadequate as a daughter, placing my father into a care facility for the first time. I didn't have any way of knowing what my rights were, nor my choices, for that matter. I wish there had been

a family 'handbook' for me. It would have avoided the many confrontations with staff that ended with them saying to me, 'Why didn't you order restraints' or "Why didn't you request information.' I just didn't know how to be my Dad's patient-advocate. I had to learn the hard way. Nursing home staff cannot expect us novices to know these things. This is a new experience for us."

Sibling Disagreements

Often adult-child caregivers find themselves in direct opposition with their siblings, and/or other family members, regarding care decisions. The direct caregiver sometimes has difficulty in relating the stress and reality of caregiving that is presenting itself. The conflict is even greater if the non-caregiving family members live a distance away and are not only NOT involved in direct care, but feel they can give sound advice without adequate understanding of the reality of the situation. Often the person with Alzheimer's disease can cleverly "disguise" his or her illness on the telephone, thus presenting a picture of a perfectly sound, aware adult. This forces the primary caregiver with the struggles of presenting a true, realistic picture of the digressing situation to siblings who are in denial.

A frustrated daughter-in-law, whose husband's siblings live far away, expresses her frustrations in this way:

"I wish her other children understood we weren't making up stories about their mother's behavior. They spoke with her rarely, yet talked to us often. Well, I finally had enough, and yesterday I let them talk with her. Her daughter hasn't stopped crying. They don't wan t to face it. They live 1500 miles away and don't live in this everyday. They just don't have a clue how hard it is!! I'm up tonight with my mother-in-law. She told me she is waiting for her boyfriend to get back from Japan. Guess he went off to war. Who knows?!"

One sibling offers this suggestion to family members:

"If you don't fully understand the situation because you 'talked

on the phone to Dad and he seems OK to me,' I have this to say: Come into town and stay with Dad for ONE week. I can almost guarantee within three days, you, my dear sisters and brothers, will realize the complexity and seriousness of the situation of Dad living alone."

"My 85-year-old mother-in-law who has Alzheimer's disease is living with my husband and me, and she seems to be regressing VERY slowly," laments this family caregiver. *"I wonder how many years she will be here and if I'll be able to cope. My brother-in-law and his wife live just 30 minutes away from us and I find my self resenting their freedom to go out, to travel, and just have time alone together. It's extremely difficult for me to understand why we have to do all the primary caregiving."*

Another daughter resolves her situation this way:

"When I first heard that Mom had Alzheimer's disease I thought that her death would come quickly. I was wrong about that, but I am not wrong about her prognosis. I cannot get my siblings to understand the gravity of the situation. They are all in denial and I am left with my own more realistic acceptance of our situation."

"I'm beside myself! I have to care for my step-dad, and I have no support!" cries a frustrated step-daughter. *"Even though my step-dad has four natural adult children, none of them has come to see him since all of this started five years ago. Just because he is in the nursing home does not mean he no longer needs their support. I have to act as his advocate, for there is no one else who will speak up for him. Where are his other children when he needs them?!"*

"I wish my brothers and sisters would understand caregiving in these final days is totally exhausting," one daughter voices. *"I am drained and do not think I can go on. For two weeks we expected Dad would die from his heart attack and the ensuing pneumonia. Now he appears to be reviving. How dare he!! I feel blasphemous in saying that but it is honest. Mom and I don't think we have the emotional*

and physical strength to go on—yet he does. What kind of life is he going to have? What does this agonizing death mean? He has multiple bed sores, groans in pain, has trouble breathing and swallowing. What further lessons does God expect us to learn from this? But most of all, why don't my brothers and sisters help us?" questions a family member in pain.

"The greatest stress in our situation with our elderly father (87) who has Alzheimer's disease is that he still lives alone and we, as siblings, cannot agree on what is best for him," explains one adult daughter. *"I believe dad should be in an adult care facility, my older sister does not, and my younger sister wants to please both of us so she keeps changing positions. I cared for dad a few days a week until my own health situation became serious. I could not keep this up. My sisters don't seem to understand."*

Family caregivers often have more problems with other family members than they do with the person for whom they are caring:

"My husband and I care for his 76-year-old mother who has Alzheimer's disease, among other problems. We aren't having super terrible problems with her care yet. We are, however, having problems with his brother and sister who live in another state. They don't want to know how she's doing if it'll upset them. His oldest sister asked that we not call her and tell her what Mom was doing cause it upset her. His younger sister isn't sending mom any Christmas present because Mom doesn't remember her. Is that insane? Where can I find information about families of Alzheimer's patients who live out of town or who just hand control to another child? His brother said in the beginning he would keep her six months if we kept her the first six months. She has gotten worse and now they have come up with two dozen reason why they can't keep her. They think it wouldn't be good for Mom to move because she wouldn't know them. What can we do as caretakers to get through the denial of help from her other children?"

A concerned daughter advocates for her dad this way:

"By refusing to place our mother in a long-term care facility, my sister is forcing our dad to exhaust what limited emotional resources he has left. I worry about him and she just doesn't understand."

"I wish my mother remembered that her parents, brothers, and sisters are dead and that it's not 1948," remarks another daughter. *"She lives with us now. She isn't able to do what she used to do for herself. She wears a diaper and when she forgets that she wears them, she'll take them off, wherever. Last night she 'boobooed' in her diaper and instead of calling for me (we use a baby monitor between our rooms at night), she took off the diaper and rubbed it on the wall. She forgets to eat and drink which is causing other problems. We try and try, without luck, to get her to eat. The doctors think it's so easy to just give it to her and tell her to drink. It doesn't work! I wish everybody in America was educated about Alzheimer's, especially Mom's other children who live out of state!"*

Frustration with family members who don't understand was expressed well by this caregiver:

"I wish someone would understand the feelings of helplessness I have when my sister-in-law causes problems for me and it does no good to explain. It is my responsibility to work, maintain a home, and care for someone who is harder to care for than a small child. The only time my sister-in-law was almost lucid and clear-thinking was when her sister came over for a surprise visit. The sister left our home thinking everything is fine and that all her sister's needs were being met, and that she didn't need to be put in a home."

"Just because Mom has Alzheimer's does not mean she has to be in a nursing home at this time!" emphatically states this daughter. *"I've quit my job and am doing a good job taking care of her. We go shopping, (granted I don't get much shopping done with her, but she*

is getting out and getting some fresh air and seeing the sights of the season.) and we go on little outings and have a good time. My brother and sister would have put her in a nursing home two years ago, but Mom had given me Power of Attorney for health care and I believe this is the best thing for her at this time. If the time comes to put her in a nursing home, I will do it, but not until that time! My children are enjoying their Grandma and their friends accept Grandma the way she is. I think if someone else tells me I should put Mom in a nursing home, I might explode! It's easy to say when it's not your parent or when you are not involved with the person for 24 hours a day. When Dad died, he left me to care for his most precious gift; I plan to do my best ."

Many siblings do not agree in the proper continuing care of a parent with Alzheimer's disease, adding to the frustrations of the primary caregiver. However, it is usually the siblings who live farther away, those not involved in the every day care of the parent, who seem to be in denial and lack a clear understanding of the magnitude of problems and decisions left to the direct caregiver. There is no one solution to sibling disagreements about care. Open and honest communication about the realities of the primary caregivers' feelings and ideas should take precedence over non-caregiving siblings.

Sadness and Grief

It is said the families who have a loved one with Alzheimer's disease suffer the grief of loss twice: once when the diagnosis becomes apparent, and again at the actual death of that loved one. Although there are many similarities between other diseases and the sense of loss, none are more poignant than the relentless, progressive loss through Alzheimer's disease. The bereavement process actually begins with anticipatory loss of cognitive functions, and proceeds through to the actual death of the person with Alzheimer's disease. Some people call this "anticipatory grief." It is the grief someone experiences when they imagine an illness, separation or loss. With Alzheimer's disease, this "anticipatory grief" process begins with the early onset of recognizable symptoms, sort of explodes with the actual diagnosis of those symptoms, and deepens as the symptoms worsen. Unfortunately, it is this kind of grief, <u>before</u> a person dies, that is most often misunderstood or minimized.

The need to grieve the loss even before the actual death of a person with Alzheimer's disease, and the support to do this grieving, is the key to working through that grief. With Alzheimer's families, it is important to understand a caregiver's need to acknowledge each loss as it occurs and to integrate those feeling expressed into understanding and acceptance by supportive people.

"I must learn to express the pain I hold within," rationalizes one daughter. *"My mother with whom I live and adore, is in the early stages of Alzheimer's. It is so difficult with the onset of a new year to acknowledge that she will only continue to deteriorate. I feel so helpless and my world feels very out of control. I do not want to give her up and I feel like that is what this disease is asking me to do. Although I am very aware others are experiencing the same journey, I still approach the future with great trepidation. I feel it is too early in the process to be so overwhelmed by aversive emotions, so I find myself desperately searching for control in a world I cannot control. Although I have a sister who is helpful, I, by choice and emotional makeup, am my mother's primary caretaker and therefore, feel the need to be "strong". I would like to discover that gray area which will allow me to maintain some degree of emotional health as we wander down this road riddled with bumps and potholes. I am so sad because I know how this story ends."*

One loving caregiver advises the following:

"Do your grieving at your own pace. It takes a lot of time to heal the wounds created by Alzheimer's disease. If you need help with

the grieving or the guilt, please seek out those who can help. There is no shame in asking for help."

Other family caregivers lament their sadness and grief in these words:

"The worst part was watching my father go from a large six-foot-four man to a skinny man who looked like a concentration camp victim."

"I grieve more each time I watch my father's memory of different things begin to fail, and see him wandering and forgetting where he is."

"The saddest thing was when my father became paranoid and convinced that everyone was after his money. I see this gentle, loving man become withdrawn and hateful, and I die a little more."

"The worst part for me was when my Dad was unable to speak and make me aware of his pain. The pain I feel is so deep."

"The saddest thing is that my dad died suddenly. Then Mom was diagnosed with Alzheimer's disease just three months after his death. After 42 years of supporting each other, my mom now has to face this diagnosis without his loving support, and my sister and I do, too. He was only 65; she is 64."

"My dad died recently, and now my Mom has Alzheimer's disease. I have lost my dad, and now I've lost my mom, too. She will never be the person she was before."

"The saddest thing is the fact that my mother does not know me anymore. She says she used to baby-sit me. I've already lost the mother I had."

"When I first heard my mother-in-law's diagnosis of Alzheimer's disease, my feelings were immediately ones of doom, hopelessness and heartache. I began my grieving almost immediately."

"With her Alzheimer's-diseased mind, Mom's abilities, memory, and her spark died first. The body only catches up later. She (my mother) is gone."

"Although my mother is clinically alive, I lost Mom months ago. It is as if she has been diagnosed with cancer or another potentially fatal disease. If another physical illness does not cause her death, Alzheimer's disease certainly will."

"Watching the person physically and mentally degenerate; watching this person lose all dignity and 'self'; the inordinate amount of care required and the loss of communication—these are what hurt the most."

"I think the saddest thing is how my Mom repeats herself over and over, not recalling she had just said what she is now telling you again."

"The worst part is to watching my father's health slowly deteriorate and knowing there is nothing that can help."

"I am now my mother's mother—no longer her daughter."

"For years my mother would call the cemetery to speak to my Dad, who died several years before. But now she doesn't even remember today is Dad's birthday. It's funny because it is just as sad today when she doesn't remember anything, as it was when she only forgot that Dad was dead. It hurts so much to see her sink into her past, and not even remember Dad was a part of that past."

"The saddest thing is my Dad survived and overcame alcoholism for 23 years, and now he and my Mom have to try to deal with his Alzheimer's disease diagnosis."

"The most frustrating thing is knowing no improvement is possible. I am devastated that I will never get my 'real' mom back."

"When I first heard my dad had Alzheimer's disease, my thoughts were 'My father is mortal.' It's funny that I never thought of that before. This diagnosis seems to slam us into reality."

"I look into my mother's dark and empty eyes and wonder where she is. Are you 10 again and going to the circus? Are you happy? Are you sad? Will you let me in for a little while? My mother

is not there—she is gone, but we will care and love the person she has become. I cannot 'fix it,' but I can be there for her."

"He's become a prisoner of his own mind," one son laments *"and I am the son who is forced to hire the warden to follow him around and keep him in line."*

A nurse professional says this:

"To me, it is a never-ending grieving process. With each new loss or new behavior, I feel and see my Mother leaving me. Even with my professional knowledge base, I can not cease my Mother's pain and the continual loss of the essence of my MUM."

"The saddest day was the day I realized my father didn't remember who I was."

"I remember her as a super smart mother who was interested in art, painting and music. She had survived a life of extreme hardships. But now she is reduced to being the laughing stock of her friends because she tells the exact same stories, almost by rote. This makes me so sad."

"My father was a superstar at U.S. Steel for 43 years, and a proud and very athletic person. The father I knew is no longer with us. He remains only a shell of a man being kept alive on a feeding tube."

The pain, the emptiness, the sadness, and the grief caregivers experience begin with the recognition of the reality of Alzheimer's disease, and continue through the perhaps years of caring, to the final ending and struggle of acceptance. Nothing prepares these families for this journey. Loving support is the only thing that can help them along their path.

Learning Ways to Cope

Cope: to endure, to contend with, to survive.

The following adult children caregivers share their feelings as they struggle to cope with a parent who has Alzheimer's disease. They share their thoughts and ideas not only to endure, but to survive.

✗

"In relationship to my Dad, I panicked thinking about my mother's inability to cope with him. I knew this diagnosis was one with which *she* *could not cope. But could I?"* questioned one son.

"Although I don't believe I ever really accepted my Dad's illness, I learned to cope by experiencing joy when there was anything he *could* *remember,"* says another.

"After caring for my mother-in-law all day, I find it extremely important to take some time for myself when my husband gets home," comments a daughter-in-law. *"No matter what time it is, I need to go upstairs and stay for at least an hour, sometimes more. I take a book with me and read, or watch TV, or just lie on the bed and try to relax. It's important for me to have this time alone, and my husband, thank God, understands and supports my relaxation time."*

A caregiving daughter found this coping tool:

"I have been taking care of my mother for almost six years, and she is now going to an adult day care center. For the first time in a long time, I do have some freedom to spend time on my computer. I say that is my sanity, and I am serious about it. Some people think I am joking, but I'm not."

"Take care of yourself," advises this caregiver who speaks from experience. *"Don't feel guilty when you take some time for yourself; it is your only hope for your survival. Because if you, the caregiver, get ill, who will take care of your loved one?"*

"My humble non-medical opinion is that Alzheimer's disease is a very individualized disease and coping skills can be learned," shares an experienced family caregiver. *"Although there are certain characteristics of various stages, I think the environment has a very large contributory role in coping. Be flexible and don't be surprised if one day things work and the next day they don't. Go with the flow. I notice my mom does best in the morning, so that's when we schedule our fun times."*

"I believe parents with Alzheimer's disease need to know what to expect too, so we came up with one way to cope: we use a 'journal' so our parent can write about how she feels. Sometimes someone else writes or tapes her conversation for her. We believe she likes to know her old memories are worth hanging on to, as well as the new ones, if possible."

"I know first-hand that time ALONE with my husband is the most valuable coping tool I have to gain the strength I need to cope with our situation. My mother seems to be awake, no matter what time we get up or go to bed. I know this may sound silly, but we spend a little extra time in the morning in the bathroom together. We both get ready at the same time which makes it perfect for us. It's only a short time ALONE with my husband, but it's a great way to begin our day. It's the only place in the entire house my mother will not interrupt us. Privacy in the bathroom has always been a family trait! We use that to our advantage."

Most personality changes that elicit difficult or rude behavior do not have an easy solution. It tries everyone's patience when the family member with Alzheimer's disease no longer "fits in" to proper social behavior. It is often hard to remember they are not children who need scolding, but adults who have Alzheimer's disease.

"Society doesn't understand such behavior and is unforgiving," this caregiver declares. *"If we could only help others understand that our loved one is ill, perhaps we can avoid unnecessary feelings of embarrassment or shame. I pray the prayer of St. Francis daily, asking God to help me to accept the things I cannot change. It goes like this:*

'Father in Heaven above,
Please help me to accept the things I cannot change,
To change the things I am able to change,
And to have the wisdom to know the difference.'"

Two caregivers who answered the surveys offered the Twelve-Step Program as their best advice in learning to cope with the effects of Alzheimer's disease on caregivers and families:

"I have used some tools to cope and deal with this disease which I would like to share with you. It takes some work but the principles are infallible. I am a certified substance abuse counselor and also a recovering alcoholic and addict and have been clean and sober for some years now. My father has Alzheimer's disease and I used the Twelve Steps of Alcoholics Anonymous to deal with the disease. They are universal principles and come from the Bible. I am not a religious freak, but have grown spiritually over the years as a result of applying these steps to my life. I now enjoy peace and serenity where there used to be self-pity and resentment. These steps will give you a 'new pair of glasses' from which to see the world."

"One of the best helps I discovered was given to me at a support group meeting: adapting the Twelve Steps from the Alcoholics Anonymous Program to my caregiving experiences. It gives me the strength and hope I need in dealing with my family member, reminds me to seek the help of a Higher Power, and helps guide my words and actions. Here is what it says:

Twelve Steps For The Caregiver

1. *Although I cannot control the disease process, I need to remember I can control many aspects of how it affects me and my relative.*
2. *I need to take care of myself so that I can continue doing the things that are important.*
3. *I need to simplify my lifestyle so that my time and energy are available for things that are really important at this time.*
4. *I need to cultivate the gift of allowing others to help me, because caring for my relative is too big a job to be done by one person.*

5.   *I need to take one day at a time rather than worry about what may or may not happen in the future.*

6.   *I need to structure my day because a consistent schedule makes life easier for me and my relative.*

7.   *I need to have a sense of humor because laughter helps to put things in a more positive perspective.*

8.   *I need to remember that my relative is not being 'difficult' on purpose; rather that his/her behavior and emotions are distorted by the illness.*

9.   *I need to focus on and enjoy what my relative can still do rather than constantly lament over what is gone.*

10.   *I need to increasingly depend upon other relationships for love and support.*

11.   *I need to frequently remind myself I am doing the best that I can at this very moment.*

12.   *I need to draw upon the Higher Power which I believe is available to me."*

Sharing sensible information such as the Twelve Step Program can guide many caregivers in their approaches to loved ones with Alzheimer's disease. It is in understanding the "journey" that caregivers can begin following the path to coping with the stressful issues unique to this kind of care. The Alzheimer's Association has more information about the Twelve Step adaptation program and other caring and coping strategies. In addition, Chapter 14 emphasizes the value of support groups in helping caregivers to cope.

Respect and Love

Although many caregivers need to express their feelings of grief, frustrations, and pleas for understanding, several took the opportunity to support their feelings of continuing love and respect for the very souls of that parent they continue to hold dear. One daughter lovingly laments:

"I wish everyone could have known my mother-in-law before she got this disease. She is such a wonderful person. She has always been there for everyone in the family in time of need. Now it's her turn to be taken care of with the love she's shown others. Hopefully I'll be able to care for her in our home right to the end."

"One thing is certain, they must always know that they are loved, supported, cherished and never abandoned," another daughter reminds others.

"The saddest time was when my father cried and begged us to take him out of the hospital after he had suffered several small strokes. He was terrified, confused, and frightened, and we couldn't help him except to assure him of our love, support and that he was safe," recalls another family member. *"These are the keys to care,"* she added.

"After losing my father to Alzheimer's disease just a year ago, and now experiencing it all over again with my mother, the thing I've learned is that we must remind them they are loved, no matter what, and that they are safe," reiterates still another caregiver.

"I make sure my mother understands that she is not stupid," this daughter suggests. *"I work to preserve her rights and her need to be treated as the individual she is, and not labeled as mentally ill. I let others know she is loved and lovable."*

"I wish I knew more exactly about the disease. I still don't know how he (my dad) was affected by it, besides that it destroyed his mind and took his life," laments a young son. *"I wish someone could tell me what it is like for someone with Alzheimer's. Not just how one feels right after diagnosis, but up until they take their last breath. Did my Dad know that he had a family and he was loved dearly?"* he questions.

A loving daughter had this to say:

"I wish my family and friends understood that caring for a dementia patient is not 'like raising a child,' as I have been told by several (my sister, an aunt, friends — none of whom are helping in

any way with my mother's care). It is much, much harder. There is no hope that Mom will improve, no chance that she will recover as the years go by. She shouldn't be reprimanded or punished when she does something wrong, for she didn't do the deed in defiance. The 'care and feeding' can't even be compared to that of a severely retarded child, for there is a level of respect that should be had for her wisdom, experience and age. On no level, other than the most basic, are there any similarities between dementia victims and children, and they shouldn't be treated as if there were!"

"The person with Alzheimer's disease has strengths and self worth even in the end stages of the disease," this caregiver learned.

Another caregiver uses Shakespeare to get her point across: *"I wish everyone would understand that even though the person has dementia, he should not have to be 'put away' or out of sight to accommodate other people's sensitivities. If I might quote Shakespeare here: 'In nature, there is no blemish but the mind. None can be called deformed, but the unkind.'"*

"I want my Dad to always know he is safe, and he is not crazy, but has a disease in his brain that is making him confused," says this daughter. *"Since he cannot understand this, all we can do is love him."*

"I love and respect my Mom so much and I try to convey this to others," a daughter comments. Her intentions are often in vain, however, as she shares this pointed comment:

"I wish people would talk TO Mom, not AROUND her. I find even the most well-intentioned people tend to ignore her, even to the point of interrupting Mom while she is talking, to ask me a question, or comment on a completely different subject. They don't even realize they do it. To them, Mom is practically a non-entity. It is a shame because, although she may not have much to say of any substance, she knows she has been ignored, and she eventually just stops talking. It breaks my heart. (And once in a while, Mom DOES have something useful to say!)"

Hopes

Adult children caregivers, in the face of caring for a parent with Alzheimer's disease, also share several comments about their hopes and determinations:

"Any improvement in my mother's condition, no matter how small, is important. I believe a lack of deterioration is an improvement!" states another daughter defending her optimism.

"We all need to understand there still can be some quality of life for our loved one, no matter what stage of Alzheimer's disease they are in.," says another hope-filled family caregiver.

"There are rewards," points out another caregiver. *"The most obvious one is knowing in your heart you are giving love that no one else is willing to give at a time when it is most important. Those who avoid being around Mom because it is 'uncomfortable' or because it is 'awkward' are missing out on a unique opportunity. My mother's sense of humor has become quite delightful; at times she is quite impish and enjoys it immensely. I love her for it!"*

In a recent Associated Press article dated September 5, 1997, former President Ronald Reagan's son, Michael Reagan, had this to say about his "rewards":

"Alzheimer's disease has robbed my father of most of his ability to speak. You can't really carry on a real conversation with him anymore. I try to talk with him at his own level. He cannot have a conversation, but he knows who we are. That's good enough for me."

Lessons Learned

Some adult caregivers, especially after their parent passes away, begin to look back and reflect on what their caregiving experience has taught them. They reflect on what many psychologists try to get people to do: live in the present moment.

"I believe God put persons with Alzheimer's disease in our world to teach us the lesson of the importance of living in this single present moment," this caregiver suggests. *"If you look at the severely demented person who relies entirely on another human being to care for his every need, you see a person who lives only in this precious moment of time. He fears not the future nor laments about the past, because his disease has robbed him of both functions. He trusts totally in the care he will receive in this precious present moment of time. It is an awesome responsibility for us children of parents with Alzheimer's disease."*

A devoted daughter, who tries hard to let her mom do the things she can still do, sums it up this way, *"Alzheimer's disease is a terribly painful disease, but it has taught me to slow down and enjoy life. I live my life more from the heart now."*

"Alzheimer's is a terribly painful disease, yet I believe it teaches us lessons," comments another family member. *"It has certainly taught me to slow down, take time to smell the roses, and enjoy my life. It is a new way of living from the heart, rather than the head.*

"The pain of Alzheimer's disease has taught me to be much more patient with everyone and to consider what might be going on in the other person's head and heart before I react to their actions and words," remarks an experienced caregiver.

"The one thing I want people to know," says one daughter-in-law/caregiver, *"is to please remember 'there, but for the grace of God, go I.' You too could end up being a caregiver or the patient. Put yourself in those shoes before you assume, judge or VOTE. You may not be in this position today, but the statistics say chances are pretty good you or someone you love will be a caregiver some day!"*

A caregiver/daughter-in-law adds this statement:

"Also know there are positives to this situation, although sometimes I have to look pretty hard to find them. I do consider caring for my parent as a growth experience."

Another caregiver expresses her thoughts this way:

"When I attempt to think through my caregiving experience, my brain becomes numb. I think the numbness is a defense mechanism against an experience that cost me my job, almost cost me my marriage, and put me into clinical depression and counseling. But I am determined to become a better person because of this. My passionate desire is to help other caregivers through my experience. I am in the process of changing careers, inspired in part by my experience with my mother. My passionate desire now is to help educate other caregivers through my experience. Educating the public is one way to accomplish this."

Conclusion

One survey from a daughter in her early fifties, quite innocently started off as an expression of her feelings, and literally turned into a compassionate, though desperate letter to her Mom. It is shared here in its entirety, for two reasons: one, to thank this caregiver for sharing her deep feelings; and two, to help all to understand the depth of frustration and pain of being a parent to a parent:

"I wish my mother understood that I love her, and I am trying to do the best I can for her. I am taking permanent guardianship, which is a thing no child should have to face: getting total control of 100 percent of a parent's affairs. When the process is complete, she will have no civil rights, no legal identity, no discretionary powers of her own, will not be able to vote, to sign legal documents, to dispose of her own money, to drive a car, or to do anything else adults are allowed to do in America.

"This is a terrifying responsibility. I get to say whether she lives at home or in a nursing home. I get to decide if she falls ill whether they treat the illness aggressively or just try to keep her comfortable until she dies. I get to decide how her hard-earned, long-

saved money is spent. I get to pick her doctor, her medication, her caregivers.

"I promise, Mom, that I will do my best to do for you as you would have wanted me to when you could make choices, but I am not really clear on what choices you would have made. You wanted to live out your life at home, but now you refuse help that could allow you to do that without starving to death or living in filth. You wanted 'no extraordinary means' applied when you came to the end of your life, but is hospitalizing you for dehydration and starvation an extraordinary means?

"You wanted to finish your days with Dad, but now you curse him and call him unbelievable names, which makes it impossible for him to care for you. You also said you'd rather be dead than 'be a burden.' I love you, Mom, but your resistance to care is making you a burden in a way you could not have foreseen. We both would care for you with great tenderness, if only you would allow it. I miss the YOU that used to be so alive! I try to hold that person in my mind always. I love you. I'm sorry."

Adult children caregivers have spoken out. They have shared their innermost feelings about frustrations, fears, guilt, grief and love. The ability of the adult child to change attitudes and reactions to situations involving a parent, is the only way to reduce the tension and struggles of that present parent-child relationship. Once an adult child can overcome past feelings, a new relationship with a parent can be formed. The determination to build a whole new relationship with a parent who now has Alzheimer's disease may make a difference in one's ability to cope.

J. Michael Dolan's book entitled "How to Care for Your Aging Parents... And Still Have a Life of Your Own," is one source of information which looks at the realities of caring for a parent. His compassionate understanding of even the most guilty thoughts and feelings of adult-children when the stress of caregiving for their elderly, demented parent takes its toll, is comforting and reassuring, and validates the existence of such sometimes irreverent thoughts.

Additional sources of information to help in the caregiving of parents can be found in Angela Heath's book "Long Distance Caregiving," "How to Care For Your Aging Parents, A Handbook for Adult Children" by Nora Jean Levin, and "Seven Steps to Effective Parent Care" by Donna Cohen. More information is listed in the Resources cited at the end of this book.

8
YOUNG PEOPLE SPEAK OUT

Alzheimer's disease is most often associated with the elderly, but young people are frequently the "silent victims" of this disease personally or through relationship. Today more and more people are being diagnosed with Alzheimer's in their early fifties or even younger. Whether it is a younger person who has Alzheimer's disease himself, a young family caring for loved one with the disease, or a grandchild struggling to understand the meaning of this cruel disease, there is no doubt that Alzheimer's disease affects everyone in the family.

One man speaks up for himself and tells of his personal anger and frustration in today's "system" which does not accept a younger person with Alzheimer's disease:

"At age 53, I myself have been tested and found to have dementia, possibly early Alzheimer's. I have requested disability and have been denied, mostly because my employer reported that he did not notice anything wrong with me. I am no longer employed by them (cut backs), but cannot collect unemployment compensation because my doctor reports to them I cannot work. I can't get disability because the state says I can still work (I taught at a tech college.) This has been so hard on my wife and myself, causing me even more confusion and anger."

Younger adult children share their views on how caring for a parent with Alzheimer's disease has turned their lives into turmoil:

"I feel that most people around me think I have a 'good grip' on things because I am young," relates one lonely daughter, *"but they just don't realize what a thin thread I am hanging by. Because my mother had Alzheimer's disease for so long, people naturally think I*

just 'get used to it.' In reality, let me tell you, there are many various phases a caregiver must continue to go through. I feel very alone."

"I wish I had known that Alzheimer's can strike so early. My mother was diagnosed at 52. Her care has turned our lives up-side-down. It is NOT just an 'old person's' disease," laments this family member.

"I wish my friends and co-workers understood it is just as hard for the caregiver as it is the Alzheimer's patient," remarks a young caregiver. *"Sometimes I feel like I have Alzheimer's disease myself. I must live with memories that I find on paper, in photographs, smells, and miscellaneous items that remind me of a time when that person was 'whole.' These items remind me of a time when my mother had dreams, aspirations, and could give back. Now I take care of her. When other people my age (mid-thirties) are raising children, I am taking care of my young mother and her finances, health, and well-being. Although she is in a rest home, I still must spend a lot of time making sure her needs are met and that she is being treated fairly. I am a single, only-child, and I feel that some of my best years have been spent taking on this depressing responsibility."*

A young woman in her twenties expresses this plea:

"I wish my mother, knew that I love her! It is very hard for me to watch my mother disappear before my eyes, and there is nothing I, or anybody else, can do about it. My mother is only 54 years old. My father is 53, however he looks 60. I'm losing my mother; he is losing his 'life.' I sometimes want to take care of him, more than my mother. That sometimes makes me feel guilty. My mother is still at home and able to do many things, but there are many things she cannot do. My father, through special planning, has been able to send my mother to day care. It makes me sick to think there are many others out there who do not have the money or the support from family. When will the government and insurance companies see this is a growing disease!!

Thank you for allowing me to share. I could say so much more!"
Another loving daughter shares her sadness:
"The most heart-wrenching thing I remember is my Mom, who has early Alzheimer's disease, saying to my Dad with great sadness regarding the future: 'There won't be any ME left.'"
"At 27 years of age, I am the youngest daughter of my 66-year-old Dad who has Alzheimer's disease. It's hard for me to reconcile the man who cannot feed himself with the 'Giant' from my childhood who danced with me on his shoulders," ponders another daughter.
"I am only 26 years old and have terrible guilt because I have taken over my 73-year-old father's life," this caregiver explains. *"I feel as though my life is out of control. I resent when people shrug their shoulders and say 'It's only memory loss!' Don't they understand that it takes away the person you once knew and leaves someone with the mentality of a child!"* she implores.

Young Families Tell Their Stories
So often when Alzheimer's disease is discussed, it is the elderly with mature adult families that come to mind. It is equally important to recognize the impact of this disease on young families struggling for understanding in today's society. The following narratives portray the concerns and confusion of young families dealing with the personal care of their loved one.
"My Mom's schedule doesn't conform to the schedules of most young families like ours. The activities, number of people, noise and surroundings in normal homes like ours, will worsen her condition by increasing stress as the disease progresses. We are at a loss as to what to do " relates one wife and mother as she reveals her conflict.
A daughter-in-law shares about the impact of Alzheimer's disease on her family:
"I wish everyone would understand that taking care of my mother-in-law is very, very challenging. It takes all I have to take care

of her. It is a terribly sad thing because everyday I see her slipping further and further away. My husband and I have moved ourselves and our three young children from our own home into my in-laws' house to help care for them. We had to modify their home to fit all of us. Now I take care of them completely. I do all of the shopping , cooking, cleaning, errand-running, child care, and elder care. My father-in-law has emphysema. He treats my mother-in-law as if she were a child. He scolds her for silly things, like when she doesn't understand, or if she cries. Both of my in-laws have found it very difficult to adjust to my children. They scare my mother-in-law. My father-in-law says they just make too much noise. My children also have found it very difficult to cope with their grandparents. Their grandmother often rips up their homework or accuses them of killing the dog (when they were only playing). I am running out of room, so I will simply say that my life has completely changed. I now feel as if I am mother to five children instead of three. I feel so alone and welcome any help I can get."

"Sorry but I feel like I'm ready to explode most of the time," apologizes this young mother. *"I have a young family I'm trying to care for, and a dad who needs me to be his voice at the nursing home, and a full time job. I just cannot handle it any more!"*

Another young daughter-in-law adds:

"This disease not only takes away the patient's standard of living, but also that of those who have to care for the patient. By this I mean Alzheimer's has not only robbed my father-in-law of a productive future, but it has robbed my husband, myself and our young children of the freedoms most families our age have. We can't just go away any more and we always have to put him at the top of our priorities list. No decisions are made without putting his needs first. At my age of twenty-five, that is hard to deal with."

"When I first heard my mother's diagnosis, I screamed, 'NO!

That is for OLD people!' Mom is only 52!! How can I tell her I am pregnant when she won't be around to see my child graduate?" cries a distraught mother-to-be.

"I wish I had known earlier that Alzheimer's disease was a possibility in my young (65-year-old) mother," voices another family caregiver. *"She had been treated for years for depression, to no avail. Her doctors never mentioned the possibility that it might be Alzheimer's disease. An earlier diagnosis would have saved us so much frustration as a family."*

"The saddest thing that happened was the day I realized Mum couldn't live with us any longer," recalls this wife and mother. *"My sons aged 13 and 16 had almost permanently isolated themselves in their room, so as not to have to deal with their confused grandmother. My husband and I couldn't get any sleep as Mum wandered up and down the hall in her high heels night after night. Everything was getting lost in the house, including Mum. It was the hardest thing for me to do, to have to decide the next step in the process. I struggle with thoughts about who needs me more, and how can I be a dutiful, loving daughter, wife and mother all at the same time."*

"I love my job, and I feel guilty that my company and coworkers are so supportive of my responsibilities to my mom," states a working mom. *"It doesn't often interfere with my work, but occasionally it does. I feel a daughter's responsibility of caring for my 82-year-old mother and feel guilty that I can't always be there for her daily needs. It is a definite 'catch 22.' I also feel I have placed a great burden on my sons by having to have their grandmother live with us. I am very lucky my 19-year-old son who lives at home, works full time, and is going to college in the evenings, is never resentful of her and helps me as much as he can. My older son lives in another state and he helps when he is here. They both have that childlike belief their mom can do anything! I question my own capabilities."*

Not all comments from young families were regretful. The following caregiver relates her anger with others who don't understand her total commitment:

"My children are enjoying their Grandma and their friends accept 'Grandma' the way she is. I think if someone else tells me I should put Mom in a nursing home, I might explode! It's easy to say when it's not your parent or when you are not involved with the person for 24 hours a day. When Dad died, he left me to care for his most precious gift: my mother. I plan to do my best, <u>together</u> with my young family."

Teenagers Pledge Their Love

When this reply came in from a 17-year-old young man, a special category was created for teenagers whose parent has Alzheimer's disease. It is hard to imagine the depth of the feelings as he writes:

"I wish my Mother knew how much I love her. She developed Alzheimer's pretty early. She's now only 52 and almost all of her cognitive skills are gone. All she does now is walk around and make noises. Her vocabulary only consists of about 12 words. I wish she would understand that I love her no matter what condition she's in. I know I'm young, and I'm not the primary caregiver; my father is. I'm only 17, but I do as much as I can for my mother.

He continues, *"I've been doing a little research on the topic, and I found your site on the Internet. I thought maybe my input could help, even though you're probably getting tons of responses. From the viewpoint of a high school student, it's really hard having a mother with Alzheimer's disease. Friends have really no idea what's going on and it's hard to explain it sometimes. It's hard not having my mother there to motivate me in my studies, college pursuits, and activities. Usually it's the mother who does most of that, since my father works.*

✄

"It's also hard to watch my father struggle," he relates. *"I can't imagine how it feels to have the woman you love and vowed to spend the rest of your life with, just crumble, and knowing that there's nothing you can do. For me it's gotten to the point where it's really hard for me to imagine when my mother was 'normal'. But it's something I accept. I want her to know that I'm here. I want to know what's going through her head. I want to know a lot. But I can't. I hope this helps."*

What courage and maturity for such a young person! It is certain that his mother feels his love and respect.

A young college student writes, *"The most frustrating thing about this disease is my friends don't understand why I go home every weekend from college and what is really happening to my dad. They do not seem to understand he is still a person and we cannot treat him like he is not there. I wish someone could have warned me about how ignorant people can be so rude and heartless when it comes to dealing with the victims of Alzheimer's disease and their families. I've learned the hard way."*

Another college student whose Dad has Alzheimer's disease relates this sad observation:

"My Dad is being treated so hurtfully by the so-called 'friends' we thought we had. It is so sad when he forgets the little things that were just told him. So his friends don't come by much any more."

A teenager sadly conveys her interpretation:

"I am watching my mother's eyes transform from the mother I once knew, into those of a complete stranger."

The following teen requests more support from the family physician:

"I wish doctors understood how much we need support as a family with young children. They should give information to us on area support groups. They need to help us when there are young children who need support also."

"My Dad needs to know we are here for him and will not leave him," states another teen. *"He needs to know there are support groups for him and us as a young family dealing with this disease."*

"I would get so angry and frustrated with my mother and yet love her so much," defends a young adult. *"When my Dad first told me of her diagnosis I started screaming 'Why is this happening to us? What did I do wrong?' She is only 45—I'm only 19!"*

"I constantly have to remind myself that there is support out there. And that it's not anybody's fault that Mom has Alzheimer's disease even though she is still so young. I am learning to accept there will be days of extreme bitterness, and that's OK!" offers another struggling family member.

"I dread the day that will come when my Dad has no memory left and will forget us forever," laments one teen.

"It's so hard seeing this happening to my dad. But as I look at it, he's still my Daddy. It breaks my heart to know that when I get married next year, he won't walk me down the aisle. But he'll be there in my heart," a future bride promises.

"My mother has Alzheimer's disease and I am only 19," says this daughter. *"The most frustrating thing about it is suddenly having to switch roles. It is like I am now the parent and she is the child. I know she will never get to be at my wedding, at least not the way she would have if she were normal, nor will she ever really be a grandmother to my kids. I hate that she was robbed from her life, and so I must lose out on an incredible person who is also one of my best friends."*

The following two teen-agers share their personal grief and love:

"She asked me who was the oldest of her children. That's me. My heart broke into another small piece, but I will love her forever."

"I would get so angry and frustrated and yet still love her so much it hurts."

"I want others to understand that even people who are 45 like my Mom can get Alzheimer's disease. It's not just an old person's disease," remarks another teen-ager.

With wisdom and maturity this young person states:

"The general public needs to know that Alzheimer's disease is not a normal part of aging. If one in four families are affected by it, it amazes me that more people are not aware that they too can be affected. Any one of us can become a victim like my dad, who has Alzheimer's disease, and myself, who is already grieving my loss."

Grandchildren Share Their Grief

Many grandchildren of all ages answered the survey in support of their grandparents who have Alzheimer's disease. They scold, plead and pledge their support and love, even through the confusion of trying to understand. In their own words, grandchildren share their intimate feelings about a grandparent who has this disease.

Their Sadness and Pain:

"I want to know what Grandma is thinking . . . and I don't want her in frustration. I want a grandmother again. It is so sad that she can't live in her house anymore. She is stuck in a nursing home. It also frustrates me that a lot of my family members have just abandoned her. Her own children who live close don't even visit her. I just don't buy their excuse that 'it's too hard to accept.' These children of hers don't seem to have any feelings. They just don't care enough. Nothing has ever really been told to me. Grandma was hospitalized on my dad's birthday last year and from there went to a nursing home. I still don't understand this thing called Alzheimer's disease."

"The saddest thing for me is watching my Grandma at times attempting to turn on the oven, as she did for 70 years before this became a problem, and now not having a clue about how to do that task."

🎗

"It breaks my heart when I see my grandpa cry sometimes when we are talking or just when I am there. I can tell he gets sad about things and he misses me. He's like this when my grandma visits too. I feel so sad, especially when I have to leave him, and especially at night when I think of him at the nursing home and not at home with grandma, where he belongs."

"Grandpa always asks me where my sister is, when she had been away at college for over a year."

"It was so sad when my Grandpa was at a store with Grandma and he did not know who she was and he went off searching for his bedroom. Then at another time he did not know his own niece at her wedding," relates a young person.

"I was about 10 and I remember my dad telling me that my Grandma had Alzheimer's disease. She had left the stove on and was forgetting other things, too. Then she had a heart attack about a year later. It was so sad to see her decline so fast."

"At first I thought my Dad had said she had 'Old-timers disease,' so I thought it was when people got old and just started to forget things. I was not prepared for the devastation of watching my grandmother decline from an active, healthy person, to a bedridden OLD woman who did not recognize me."

Grandchildren observe and comment on the chaos and confusion within their families:

"I think the saddest thing has been watching my caretaking family members try to cope with my Grandma, who cannot even remember my name any longer."

"I remember hearing all the bits and pieces which I knew to be associated with Alzheimer's Disease (or some related dementia) and then their talking about my Grandmother. Even my family who did the hands-on caretaking did not at first know this was the diagnosis. We were devastated!"

"I wish someone would have told us earlier that my grandfather could be at financial risk, so that we could have made some personal and financial preparations for the potential onslaught that occurred in the care of my grandmother who has Alzheimer's disease."

"I remember the time Grandmother gave one of us a birthday card which wasn't addressed or signed. It was just the beginning of her forgetfulness, but it was so sad to think that she was losing her memory."

"The saddest day was when my Grandmother brought a birthday card for my father and it was not even signed. I had to sign it for her. I think she forgot it was her own son's birthday. I will always remember this as the beginning of the end of the grandmother I once knew."

"The saddest thing was when my grandfather did not even know my name. I watched it totally wear down my grandmother. My grandfather would worsen every time I saw him. He was not the same person I once knew. He would whistle at the nurses as they walked past his room, and this would embarrass my grand- mother. He got so bad I could not even bring myself to visit him. It was so sad for me."

"My grandmother, who has always been more like a mother to me, suffers from Alzheimer's disease. My mother and I had to make a lot of the decisions about what we should do and how we should handle dealing with her. That was the hardest part. My grandmother's disease has progressed very rapidly. She was diagnosed with it only two years ago. She is now in a nursing home because we cannot care for her at home. She no longer walks, she is on a feeding tube, cannot do anything for herself anymore, and basically doesn't know who we are most of the time. I think the worse thing is she is no longer the person we knew, but now like a child. The strong, vital woman we once knew as grandma, is not there anymore. All that is there is her

shell. We try to make the best of it though. We go to see her all of the time. We are very involved in the nursing home as well. I am currently president of the family council. All this helps us more than we could help her."

"I do not think people can ever fathom the pain Alzheimer's patients and their families go through. People do not realize how bad it is until someone in their family gets Alzheimer's disease. The only way you can see that kind of pain is to go through it yourself. To see my grandmother forget how to walk, how to talk, how to eat, how to go to the bathroom, forget the people she once loved , and then forget how to breath, is the most devastating kind of pain a family can endure. It is like death, without one dying".

Their Frustrations:

Grandchildren continue to share their frustrations and feelings about their relationships with a grandparent who has Alzheimer's disease:

"The most frustrating thing is attempting to relate logically and as if my Grandpa with Alzheimer's is able to respond logically. It doesn't work!"

"I wish someone had told my family and me earlier about the fact that lots of materials are available through the ADRDA (Alzheimer's Disease and Related Dementias Association) or similar organizations. They really helped us with understanding Grandpa's disease."

"Sometimes I can laugh with the rest of the family when I see Gram do funny things. Once she was shopping with my aunt and all she did was go around and fill the cart with anything she could grab, not anything she needed. It was really funny, the shopping and all. I guess you had to be there to get a laugh, and to try to see the humor in a pathetic situation."

"The most frustrating part is attempting to relate logically to my Grandma and as if she were able to respond logically."

"The worst part was when it came to a stage where I could not

even see my grandfather. He could not remember who I was. My mom and dad say that my grandfather is going to die soon."

"My grandma accused my grandfather of not feeding her and abusing her. We didn't know who to believe at first."

"Grandma often starts crying and tells me she hopes it will get better, but it only gets worse."

"Knowing there is nothing I can do to help my grandma, is the saddest thing. She seems so alone, yet I feel so helpless."

"The worst part is knowing it's only going to get worse. There is no cure, nothing to stop the degeneration."

"I wish others would understand the frustration and embarrassment it causes my grandma when they are all ridiculing her."

Another granddaughter said, *"I've found guilt is also a big thing our family has had to deal with. Questions such as: Why didn't we recognize it earlier? Is there something more we could have done? In the end, were they aware how much they were loved, even though they don't recognize us?"*

"The most frustrating thing about Alzheimer's disease is not being able to communicate with my grandmother anymore. She has no clue how to speak any longer. I just wish someone would have told me that she would lose control of all her functions like this. One funny yet heartbreaking thing that happened was when she gave me a whole stack of Band-Aids and told me they were 'good' for me! But the saddest memory I have was when my grandmother was trying to talk about her family and her only living brother. She just couldn't get the words out and she started to cry. It broke my heart again."

Grandchildren Struggle To Understand

A granddaughter in her mid-twenties has this message for her family:

"I wish the rest of the family would understand Grandma is not 'a shell of a woman,' as they all say. Her dementia has made it

only harder to see the wisdom of her age. I know she is still the loving, caring, wise and strong woman she has always been. I wish they could understand how to love her and they knew feeling their love is all she has to root her in this world, so completely unfamiliar to her now. I wish they would see my response as primary caregiver is not merely sentimental, nor is it easy. I wish they knew I need their help, their love, and their emotional support, too. I have a lot of wishes, and could ramble on all night. I just wish the whole world could be comfortable with listening—and seeing the truth as it is."

A young adult grandchild offers this plea:

"I wish all people would understand Alzheimer's disease is a disease which robs the victim of all aspects of who they were. It's an incredibly devastating process for our family to watch Grandma deteriorate into such a helpless and dependent state. In the end, we can only hope for death to come quickly to end hers and our unbelievable suffering."

"My Grand Pa sometimes forgets where he is or who I am. He has this terrible disease I don't understand. Sometimes I wonder who might get it and at what age it might begin to take its toll on the victim. I ask how to slow down its effects and to accept that this terrible disease is unstoppable for now."

Another granddaughter says, *"It is just such a shame to see Grandma like this because she has always prided herself on her intelligence and independence. I am having a hard time understanding this."*

"The most frustrating thing about Alzheimer's disease is watching an active, caring individual like my grandmother, deteriorate in increments," this grandchild explains. *"The good and bad days occur at unpredictable intervals, which may leave little recovery time or 'breathing room.'"*

"I wish someone would have told me that she (my grandma) could die from Alzheimer's disease," this grandchild laments.

✗

"My grandmother gets jealous of my stepmother, thinking my dad is my grandfather and my step-mother is 'the other woman,'" a grandchild tries to explain. *"She often would have periods of going back in time and this doesn't make sense to me."*

A granddaughter in her early twenties writes simply, *"I wish other family members would see it's not easy and I need help!"*

"She keeps forgetting my grandfather passed away and every once in a while she has to go through the pain of losing him all over again," relates this grandchild.

"I noticed something was different about my grandma when I saw her walking down the staircase backwards with high heeled shoes and pajamas on. She was also completely made up and had toilet tissue around her head. At first I thought she was just trying to be funny. Then I realized how sad it was. It was so unlike her! She would be so saddened if she realized what she was doing," remarks a caring family member.

"Sometimes it makes me uncomfortable watching people attempt to relate to my grandma, and not wanting to admit something is different or wrong. No one quite knows what to say," admits this young person.

"I heard that eventually the difficult part will be over for a person who has Alzheimer's disease (or so I assume, although I have not been diagnosed myself)," writes a granddaughter as she sorts through the facts. *"Easy to assume for someone else, I suppose. It appears that the person eventually does not experience distress. However, that's not the case for the rest of our family."*

"She was diagnosed in 1991. I remember symptoms a year earlier. I thought that word was 'Old-timers' disease, so I thought it was when people started to forget things," another granddaughter recalls.

The following family members struggle with trying to discover the right things to do:

"The entire family does not want to recognize the needs of my grandmother," states a concerned family member. *"My grandmother's husband is 80 years old and I feel is not able to care for my grandmother to the degree that is needed. I think they are both too old to care for each other and need additional help."*

"First, it is hard as a grandchild raising my own family, to step in and take over without hurting other family members' feelings. Second, I feel uncomfortable going into their home which is not the home I visited growing up as a child. I think this is one of the major obstacles for the family."

"Maybe if my grandmother's doctor would explain to the family it is time that another family member takes over washing the clothes, doing the shopping, etc., this would eliminate hard feelings between family members."

"I think patients should be told about their disease so they can make decisions for the future. My family never wanted to tell my Grandmother. They said that early in life my Grandmother stated that she didn't ever want to know if she became struck with cancer, Alzheimer's, or other debilitating diseases. Now that she has Alzheimer's disease I guess she will never know. I question the wisdom of that."

A teen-aged grandchild longs for this deeper understanding:

"I wish society understood Alzheimer's disease is not something that can continue to be shoved under the carpet. I wish everyone was able to comprehend the fact that it affects everybody. And I wish there was no need for them to have to understand that fact."

Facing Fears

Grandchildren are forced to face the reality of a disease that is so hard to understand. Here is what they expressed about their own fears:

"When I first came to realize the diagnosis of my grandma, I believe I felt sad that my family would have to endure the process. And I felt scared for my grandmother and me," admits this young person.

❧

"I first realized Grandpa had Alzheimer's disease when I picked up a paper with all the symptoms to the disease and realized he had all the symptoms. Then I thought, 'oh my God, am I at risk too!'" questions a young mind.

"The most frustrating thing is not knowing how long my grandma will be with us," sadly expresses another child.

Support and Love

Threaded throughout the comments from grandchildren were the dedication, love, and support that bind a grandchild and grandparent, even one who has Alzheimer's disease.

"I wish my Grandpa would understand that he is not alone. Many people have Alzheimer's. It may be a long road ahead, but there are people around who are willing to ease the burden—like me and my Mom and Dad," says a grandchild with assurance.

"My Grandma needs to know Alzheimer's disease is not necessarily a 'death sentence.' We as a family, and with Grandma's input, just need to look long and hard for a good nursing facility and do a lot of research before making any decisions. We need to always let her know she will be safe and loved."

"I hope my grandpa knows that we will always love him and be there for him no matter what, even if he gets to the point of not remembering me."

"My grandpa still makes funny faces and funny noises to entertain us like he did when we were little. He has always been so humorous. He still can make us laugh. I love him for that."

"Why has everyone given up on my GrandPa. It seems like some of them think that because he has changed so much with this disease, he isn't the same person. But I know he is, and he needs us now maybe more than ever."

"Here is the story: my Gram has died now, but before she died, like a month or two, we found out that my Gram had Alzheimer's disease. I got support and help from my family to understand what was happening. Now I wish I could help other people or children that need help with dealing with someone in the family with Alzheimer's," offers this grandchild.

"I wish my family would continue to treat Grandma as an adult who deserves their respect," criticizes another grandchild.

In closing this section in which grandchildren speak out, it is fitting to acknowledge the honesty and love of the following young people:

"I wish someone would have told me earlier that this may happen to my Grandpa. It makes me kind of regret not spending as much time with my Grandpa before he got so bad. I know he loves me no matter what, but I wish I would have known how much he loved me before. I wish I would have told him that I love him. It makes it hurt all the worse. He knows so many things that happened so long ago, and this is neat to me. I didn't think that he would remember them or that they would be as important to him as they are. I guess when you're younger you take advantage of some things. I am learning more as I grow up."

"I want to share a poem I wrote in honor of my grandmother who has Alzheimer's disease. I hope you do not mind:

A Grandchild's Poem
<u>As She Sits</u>

As she sits and stares at the clock,
Wishing and wanting for someone to stop,
Knowing her family soon will be there,
The ones who truly love her and care.
As seconds turn to minutes and minutes to hours,
She thinks of all their magical powers.
For her their visits are far too short,
But she can't wait to laugh and snort.
So she sits and waits for them to come,
Knowing it will be lots and lots of fun.

By: Stacey Cirillo"

9
CAREGIVING SPOUSES SPEAK OUT

With a growing percentage of spouses as caregivers, this chapter is dedicated to those who took the time to share their hopes, frustrations, determination, and sadness, so others may learn from their experiences. Surprisingly few spouses responded to the Internet survey from which these quotes were gathered. This may be attributed to two reasons: one, caregiver-spouses are too busy to answer such surveys; and/or two, caregiver-spouses, for the most part, are not computer users. Yet their heartfelt responses as spouses deserve our consideration.

"The most difficult thing is watching the person you once knew and loved all of your life just disappear completely, leaving a total stranger in the body of your loved one," is the way this spouse puts his grief into words.

Try to imagine: your loving spouse of some fifty years, your soul-mate, your confidante becomes a helpless person within the *body* of that once-loved person, but with none of the personality characteristics of that former person. Families who have a loved one with Alzheimer's disease truly go through the grief process twice—once with the loss of the personality of the person, and again at the death of that person.

Another spouse describes her experience using a profound comparison:

"I see my husband, who has had Alzheimer's disease for seven years now, like a walnut. It's as if someone took the two halves apart, removed all the walnut meat inside, and put the halves back together. He looks exactly the same as he did before the disease. Anyone looking at him would never know the difference. But what I have left, that I care for, is an empty shell of the man who was once my vibrant, loving husband."

✗

"The hardest part is having to watch someone you love slowly slip away to the point that you almost begin to ignore the changes," one wife explains. *"I more often notice his major memory losses while someone is visiting or we're out with old friends, when I look at him through their eyes, and I am shocked."*

Another spouse tells it this way:

"My husband is in the earlier stages of Alzheimer's disease, but I want to acknowledge the particular difficulties that Alzheimer's disease brings when it's a spouse who has it. Not that it's any easier or more difficult if it's a parent, but it's slightly different, I think. We expect our parents to get old, need to be cared for, and finally to die. There's something about watching my spouse disappear before my very eyes that has its own unique terror."

A loving husband voices his deep feelings within his story:

"I was the sole caregiver for my wife for nine years before I put her in a care facility. Since she watched her mother and her sister suffer and die from Alzheimer's disease, she threatened to kill herself when the early symptoms of her disease began to develop. However, as the disease progressed, it caused her to forget those threats. As she got steadily worse, I felt she would want me to assist her out of this world and I was sorely tempted many times to do just that. I never had the courage to do it and accept the consequences. I still feel guilty about this. So I go on visiting her at the nursing home, watching the day to day deterioration, hoping for an end to her ordeal . . . yet fearing it."

Early-Onset Alzheimer's Disease

Many younger husbands and wives reveal their pain and loneliness as their lives drastically change when having a spouse who is young diagnosed with Alzheimer's disease:

"Caring for someone with Alzheimer's disease is lonely and difficult. In 1980, at the age of 50, my husband was diagnosed with

Alzheimer's. I've watched him deteriorate since then. My responsibilities have increased and our roles have completely reversed. I've become the breadwinner and must make all the decisions now. Our friends have all deserted us."

"I wish more people would understand the implications on families and young victims is different when the person with Alzheimer's disease is young, as compared to when it is an elderly Alzheimer's victim. Most programs are oriented toward seniors and don't address the emotional impact on the younger families with school-aged children. My wife's illness has turned our young family upside down with concerns about genetics, financial destruction, mid-life and retirement plans."

So often, when the spouse is under 65, the families dismiss or cover-up obvious signs of mental deterioration. A 'fifty-something' woman who has since been diagnosed with Alzheimer's disease, writes this about her well spouse:

"He said he knew I was having trouble doing things but he thought that I would be OK. I wasn't taken seriously because I was 'too young' to have Alzheimer's disease."

Another spouse admits his grief and pain as he continues to care for his young wife who is being robbed of her memory:

"My dear wife, who is only 58 years old, is afflicted with the loathsome malady called Alzheimer's disease. Nothing but a physical shell of her remains. I have the privilege of caring for her. The hardest thing is that most of the time she doesn't even know me, yet she seems to know everyone else. We have been married for 40 years. She has been my closest friend all of our lives. I just cannot believe she would no longer know me."

"I wish my wife would understand she is not crazy, but is suffering from a memory loss," this spouse implores. *"She is so important to me. She and I are both 57 years of age and have been*

married for 37 years. She was diagnosed as having dementia six months ago. However, at her last doctor's visit, he stated she does have some cognitive reasoning and can remember some short-term items. I was advised the best thing would be to place her in a home where she would have 24-hour supervision. We could not afford to do that and I have her with me in Japan and where I am her primary caregiver, AND HANDLING IT TO THE BEST OF MY ABILITY. I have the supportive Internet caregivers to thank for that."

Dr. Franklin Cassel, in his booklet entitled "Flowers for Peggy," shares these thoughts as he reflects on the earlier stages:

"As I look back on those years, I believe the problem first showed itself as Peggy lost confidence in finding her way about in what had been familiar territory. I recall our having visited someone in the hospital and being surprised, when we were ready to leave, by Peggy's reluctance at my suggestion she meet me at the front entrance where I would bring the car. This we had done many times before. I now realize Peggy was beginning to forget her way about and was ashamed to tell me she was lost."

Feelings of Pain and Loneliness

"The loneliness is the worse for me. We had a terrific marriage and were extremely close," relates this wife. *"He still is dependent on me and I think, for the most part, is happy and content. I am the one whose life has changed and now make all the decisions alone."*

"My wife no longer recognizes me as her husband," a distraught spouse reveals. *"She thinks I am a stranger and keeps asking me, 'Where is Arthur?' Well, I am Arthur! She even asks the neighbors who I am and where is Art? It's so sad!"*

"I wish others would understand what it is like day by day to care for someone with whom you have had a sharing relationship, and who now doesn't even know you are her spouse," a sad husband relates.

Other spouses remark:

"In caring for my husband, I feel exasperated one moment and filled with guilt the next."

"How can I cope with friends and family members who deny that anything is wrong with my husband?" is a frequent cry among spouses.

"The most frustrating thing about Alzheimer's disease is the helplessness: the feeling of total frustration with the situation. There is no cure; there is no hope. There is only the day to day constant awareness of the effect it has on the quality of my wife's life, and on mine and our children."

A concerned daughter pleads with her mother who is primary caregiver for her dad:

"My Dad needs my Mom to be patient with him as he struggles with his new identity. He needs her undivided attention, her warmth, and her resolve to not argue with him as he makes mistakes or repeatedly asks her the same questions."

"My wife seems to know me when I first return from the store or something," another spouse explains, *"but within a few minutes, she is asking me who I am, and where is her husband. I feel absolutely useless because she doesn't know me or trust me and I just don't know what to do."*

Occasionally the circumstances of being a spouse/caregiver bring rewards to grateful recipients:

"I never realized how many good friends we have here where we live. I only hope there is some way I can let them know how much I appreciate all the wonderful help and love they have shown my husband and me during these tough times of caregiving. I know it will not be possible in my lifetime, but I am sure God will see they are rewarded. My family is all up north and I consider these wonderful people our 'second family.'"

❧

"I am capable of caregiving for my husband while keeping my sense humor," one wife says with conviction. *"He's in the early stages, but I am determined to help him maintain his dignity and independence for as long as possible without losing my own sense of self-worth. It's a lonely job without him though."*

Resentment

It is understandable that spouses harbor feelings of resentment and grief over the loss of the companionship of a spouse despite their loving caregiving efforts. Some had this to say:

"I keep giving and giving and still see that my caring efforts are not enough for my wife."

"The worst part for me is knowing and realizing I cannot meet the needs of my husband, and then seeing our relationship stolen by this disease. How can I continue to handle this and what lies ahead for us?"

"Alzheimer's is a hidden disease. The person who has it, particularly in the early stages, does not appear to have anything wrong with them. They are usually physically in pretty good condition, depending on their age, but mentally they are lost. I find even people who have known my husband for years still don't always see the deficits he has, because he does have a way of covering them up. It is so easy to stick your head in the sand about Alzheimer's because of this problem. It seems no matter how much I tell people about what is happening, they still don't really have a feel for what it is that the I, as the caregiver, am going through. Everyone comes up to my husband at church and says, 'My, he's doing fine!' But I keep wanting to say, 'Just come and stay with him for 24 hours and you will get a different picture, the REAL picture.' But I never say it. I just think it."

"I wish someone would have told me earlier how very difficult it would be to get information and help about the care of my wife

with Alzheimer's disease. If it were not for my computer, I would be totally frustrated. It is my link for information and even for comfort (through Chat Groups). I have struggled for three years through a maze of misinformation. And when I finally went on-line, I felt I had been saved! But everyone does not have this tool. I feel lucky to have it!"

"Somehow our spouses with Alzheimer's disease need to find the ability to enjoy what they can still do and don't worry about what they can't. They are still grownups, not children. I wish my friends would understand this."

Sharing Ideas

Spouse/caregivers express their thoughts and feelings as they share their coping ideas learned through personal experiences.

"I wish others understood this is an illness and nothing of which to be ashamed and that it makes it easier to simply share the fact of the disease with others. When they know what the problem is, that my husband has Alzheimer's disease, it reduces the stress for all concerned. This has all worked very positively for my husband and me."

"Every person with Alzheimer's disease is different in his or her manifestation of the illness. I took care of my grandmother, and now my husband. The similarities in the two account for maybe only 30 percent of all the behaviors I've seen so far, teaching me that we can't judge each other's caregiving approaches."

"It is imperative that the spouse/caregiver give <u>herself</u> or <u>himself</u> tender, loving care also."

One caregiving spouse offers this suggestion:

"My wife talks to herself in the mirror for hours. She gets so worried about her 'friends' in the mirrors she would not even eat her meals until she checked on each one. It was getting physically

exhausting for her. So, on the recommendation of my support group, I blocked off the mirrors to reduce the distractions."

A doctor whose wife has had Alzheimer's disease for several years, shares these feelings from his writing entitled "Flowers for Peggy":

"What have I learned from my experience with Peggy? To what can we give credit for her apparent good attitude and spirit in spite of complete loss of ability to create new memory, loss of recent memory, and loss of almost all of long term memory? Looking back over the years, and especially recent days, there seems to be one outstanding factor which I feel deserves credit for Peggy's responses. It is 'Flowers for Peggy' that has turned the tide. From the moment she has been in the nursing center (three full years now), she has been showered with flowers that had been grown with my tender loving care. Flowers which more importantly were symbolic of a love from my heart which I freely expressed with words many times a day and every day. Assurance of my commitment to her and my undying devotion has been a daily fare. Peggy cannot remember and needs daily reminders. I have not failed to be with her three times daily. We constantly reassure each other of our abiding love."

Another loving spouse uses this method to protect his wife's dignity:

"When I am out with my wife I carry a card, just like a business card, with the following words imprinted on it: 'Please direct your conversation to me. My companion has a brain disorder called Alzheimer's disease. Thank you.' This helps me from having to explain my wife's forgetfulness or sometimes childlike behavior, like when ordering in a restaurant. I got these cards from our local Alzheimer's Association and they are given out free to caregivers. It seems to help others to understand us."

Concern For Elderly Spouse/Caregivers

"Where can I get help? We have no family, so I cannot discuss what I should do!" These were the frantic cries of a 70-year-old male spouse, as received over the Internet. He was referred to the Alzheimer's Association to help him find assistance in his local area. These are the victims—the elderly spouses trying to care for their loved ones—trying to be stoic and strong. They are probably crying themselves to sleep at night, only to be awakened by the wanderings of their spouses. How can these elderly people in need be helped? How can they be found and informed of assistance?

Many elderly do not have the luxury of finding time to read the newspaper or watch TV, so they would not even realize there are organizations which could help them. Most are not even certain what the problem is with their "forgetful" spouse. Most would not accept help even if it was offered. Most were raised in families where they took care of their own. Imagine the helplessness, the extreme fatigue, the relentless effort it takes 24 hours a day, to care for a spouse with Alzheimer's disease, when there is no other family.

One eighty-year-old gentleman writes and asks for help, as if he had clearly thought this through:

"Instead of a nursing home where my wife is now, is there any way she could be taken care of at home and Medicaid pay for the needed help? I mean like nurses aid help. I can furnish supplies that are needed, if only I could afford a helper."

A granddaughter vents her concerns for her elderly grandparents:

"The entire family does not want to recognize the needs of my grandmother. My grandmother's husband is 80 years old and I fear he is not able to care for my grandmother to the degree that is needed. My aunt (and the only daughter) seems to blame my grandmother's husband for not keeping my grandmother clean. I think they are both too old to care for each other and need additional help, but no one will listen to me."

"I wish everyone would understand this is a disease which affects everyone close to the primary patient. It changes the lives of family members and puts an overwhelming burden on the principal caregiver, particularly if he/she is also elderly," writes an 80-year-old female spouse.

"I am unable to care for my 80-year-old wife," this worried elderly husband confesses. *"She is in an Alzheimer's care facility which costs much more than my teacher's pension provides. I have few options left!!"*

A frustrated-sounding elderly husband responds with this comment:

"Anything I do is in her (my wife's) best interests. I do understand though that she can not understand this herself, and this saddens me, as I am her loving spouse of many years."

An added concern is when the spouse afflicted with Alzheimer's disease is abusive, and the elderly well spouse fears revealing this information to family or friends:

"The saddest thing is when my elderly husband becomes violent and physically abusive to me, and later apologizes, knowing he did something to hurt me. But he doesn't remember what he did, so I have to forgive him," explains an elderly wife as she suffers the abuse as a silent victim.

One of the biggest problems facing society is the safety of elderly couples living alone and desperately trying to deal with the perplexities of illness, memory loss, and personality changes. Advisors recommend we become aware of elderly neighbors and their needs. If an elderly couple needs assistance, please notify a social service agency which could help them. Most every community has assistance available for their elderly people. Most also have an Association of Geriatric Care Managers. Some other resources are listed in the back of this book. It is up to each person to help protect the well-being of their neighbor—especially the elderly persons.

✗

Alzheimer's Association Interview With Nancy Reagan

As one of the most distinguished caregiver/spouses, Nancy Reagan has had the boldness and courage to speak out on behalf of her husband, former President Ronald Reagan. In an extended conversation with the Alzheimer's Association, Mrs. Ronald Reagan recently shared her personal thoughts on the past year. Highlights of that conversation are reprinted here acknowledging the national Alzheimer's Association as the source:

*"**Alzheimer's Association (AA):** Mrs. Reagan, why are you and your husband committed to Alzheimer's and to finding a cure?*

***Mrs. Reagan:** The truth is, we were committed to Alzheimer's way back in the early 1980's, long before it ever touched us in a personal way. As President, Ronnie supported Alzheimer's research and declared November National Alzheimer's Disease Month in 1983. Back then, Ronnie's goal was to raise the level of awareness of this cruel disease, and make people realize they shouldn't be self-conscious or embarrassed. It's a disease like any other disease. That's the message we're still trying to convey now. I suppose when an illness changes your life, it's natural to want to reach out to the many others who are suffering — to connect with them at some level. You say to yourself, 'Okay, this is happening to us, and it's frightening and cruel. Let's try to help other families.'*

***AA:** How is President Reagan doing?*

***Mrs. Reagan:** He's doing well. He enjoys going into the office everyday, playing golf, and going to church. Weekends and holidays are spent with our children and grandchildren. Ronnie's illness has, thankfully, pulled our family back together, so in some ways this ordeal has turned out to be a blessing. We've learned to appreciate each other more and our time together. I think our daughter, Patti was right when she said* *we've established a 'zone of privacy,' something I think all families create to protect one another. We're all for openness, but our family life now is sacred.*

AA: *How are YOU doing, Mrs. Reagan?*

Mrs. Reagan: *The cards and letters keep coming in from people across the country. They've been such a tremendous source of comfort to me. Some of the notes I've received are so moving and touching, while others are from people who feel totally overwhelmed and lost. I want to assure them that they're not alone in all this. I want them to know that there are support groups out there to guide them through the dark moments; that there are people who understand what they're going through.*

AA: *Why did you choose to affiliate with the Alzheimer's Association?*

Mrs. Reagan: *The Alzheimer's Association wants to defeat this cruel disease. Honestly, we can't wait any longer to step up the research. People are living longer and their well-being has to be our top priority. The Association offers people help and hope. Ronnie and I want to support that effort. If a cure can be developed, perhaps families won't have to continue losing loved ones this way.*

AA: *Does your husband support your decision to take a public role?*

Mrs. Reagan: *Ronnie encouraged me to become involved, and we both agreed that lending our name to the Institute was the right thing to do. We've been public our entire married life, you know, and if we can make a difference through our involvement, then we've simply got to do it.*

❧

__AA:__ You've gone public before with personal health problems.

__Mrs. Reagan:__ Throughout our public life, we have made every attempt to share information about our medical conditions with the media and the American people. When I had breast cancer, I spoke openly and honestly. As a result, many women wrote to me, saying that my personal story and recovery — thanks to early detection — prompted them to be tested. That's why I feel it's so important to embrace these health issues. After all, nothing speaks louder than personal experience.

__AA:__ How do you feel about the establishment of this Institute in your name?

__Mrs. Reagan:__ This Institute, which bears our name, isn't about Ronnie and me. It wasn't established to honor two people, but to serve as a symbol of hope to all those who share our dream of a cure for Alzheimer's.

__AA:__ What would you say to all those who are grappling with this disease — as a patient or a caregiver?

__Mrs. Reagan:__ Don't ever lose hope. Even when life seems bleak and hopeless, know that you are not alone."

As a post script to this interview, the TV program "American Journal," on November 20, 1997, commented that recent reports indicate that Mr. Reagan, now 87 years old, is rarely seen in public any longer, but he continues to go to the office every day and remains "a great communicator," according to his staff. "He looks great and continues to defy the years with his youthful appearance. However, we don't end up in any meaningful conversations with him any longer," they added.

X

A special thank you goes out to former President Ronald Reagan and Mrs. Reagan for speaking out about Alzheimer's disease. They probably did more for public awareness of this disease than any other famous person in recent history. When Mr. Reagan went public in 1994, the nation took notice. Caregivers who had been shunned by friends and ignored by the government, suddenly had "a leg to stand on." Their efforts made a difference, because now there was a common interest in a long-developing problem disease.

Conclusion

The impact of a *couple* which suddenly becomes a *single* bearing the burdens of a spouse's Alzheimer's disease alone has to be one of the most devastating effects of this disease. Grateful acknowledgment is given to all who took the time to share their pain in the effort to help others to understand.

10
CAREGIVERS IN NURSING HOMES SPEAK OUT

Caregivers in institutions and facilities meet extraordinary challenges when caring for persons with Alzheimer's disease. Sometimes these caregivers, whether professional, certified or volunteer, have not had formal training in the care to meet the special needs of persons with Alzheimer's disease. Their common themes of frustration and concerns, their desires for more education for themselves, the families and their staff, as well as their heartfelt love for the persons with Alzheimer's disease, are apparent in their sharings.

Professionals Speak Out To Family Members

Some of the professional staff of care facilities speak directly to family members with their pleas:

"If your parent is at a stage that he or she is experiencing forgetfulness that interferes in their lives, it is time to take charge of the situation and protect his or her well being," a professional caregiver advises. *"You are the only one who can make the decision as to the correct timing for placement of your loved ones. But please do not be totally negative about a health care facility specializing in care for persons with Alzheimer's disease. Most times the new residents will welcome the opportunity to have persons around them who are caring for their needs. Often they relax more in an environment where the demands of 'reality' are eased and no one is pressuring them to 'remember.'"*

A nurse who also has a father-in-law with Alzheimer's disease, shares this insight: *"Caregivers don't always face the realistic facts, and therefore don't accept the inevitable. Doctors need to sit down with the primary caregivers and lay out the true course of this disease. They (the patient) have done nothing to develop this terrible disease. It isn't their fault when they forget something simple. It is not their fault that they experience depression, malaise, and general lack of interest. Families need to be informed of this early on."*

"The afternoon so long ago when I first realized that my mother-in-law had Alzheimer's disease helped prepare me for my own mother's diagnosis of early-onset Alzheimer's. I work in a long-term care facility as a nursing assistant. My mom is a resident at my facility. Everyday I see the fear and confusion on the faces of the family members. They want their loved ones fixed. We cannot 'fix' them, we can only 'be there' for them. How many times have I heard, 'Dad is just a little confused. With the proper medication he will be just fine.' or 'Why is my mother in diapers?' forgetting the fact that one of the reasons their mom is at the facility is the constant bed wetting. I feel so sorry for the families because there is such limited information available for them," a nurse assistant relates.

A professional caregiver expresses her concern this way:

"I wish families understood their loved one with Alzheimer's does not have 'cooties.' I understand the grieving process is difficult for families and the person residing in a nursing home often does not have the same personality he did prior to the disease. I also know these people and the staff who care for them need support from families, emotionally and in practical matters."

One caregiver shares this observation from her work at a care facility:

"I wish families understood that visiting your loved one is important. He or she may not know you are there when you visit, but may remember later, during a lucid moment. What they will remember is that you <u>HAVEN'T</u> visited them. Which would <u>you</u> prefer?"

"As a nurse caregiver, I wish my patients' families understood

🎗

that Alzheimer's disease is a life long illness with a forward progression. So many waste time and energy on 'wishing the disease away.' It is so sad. Medical advancements are being made every day, but may only be palliative and not curative. We need to be patient and understanding with our patients' loved ones and, yet, at the same time, we need to be 'in tune' with our own needs. Being a caregiver is not easy and staying positive for our patients' families is even harder. But don't give up on them!"

A social worker has this advice, *"One of the most difficult things for a family with a loved one with Alzheimer's disease is to assess when the risks outweigh the benefits of keeping that loved one at home. There comes a stage when a person clearly can no longer stay by himself. Each family has to determine its own acceptable level of risk. If in doubt, ask your Alzheimer's Association to recommend an agency that will come out and do a sort of safety audit to make recommendations for making the house safer for your loved one, or to recommend placement in an assisted living facility."*

A nurse comments, *"Residents with Alzheimer's disease are the same persons as before the onset of the disease. That person 'acts' differently as the disease progresses. I agree that it is very traumatic for relatives to see this change, but the person once known to the family is still 'in there' somewhere and still needs the family to accept and love them just as they did before the onset of the disease."*

A volunteer staff member says, *"It breaks my heart watching family members refuse to accept a diagnosis of Alzheimer's disease. They struggle to keep their loved ones in reality with questions to them like 'Well, you remember that, don't you?' or 'You know you just had your dinner.' Then I watch the disappointment and conflict on the faces of both the family members and the poor dementia person who doesn't remember these things."*

"For some families, the grief and the feelings of guilt become unbearable. Some who put their parents or spouse into extended care rarely visit. It is not because they no longer love their dear one. It's just that they cannot bear the pain of seeing the one they love not recognize them. Or perhaps they see themselves in a similar state in another twenty years," justifies another care provider.

Frustrations, Problems and Concerns

Several professional caregivers shared their views about the frustrations of housing persons with Alzheimer's disease and other dementias together with the mentally alert in care facilities:

"One of the most frustrating things about working as manager of a 55-bed special care unit within a 300-bed, restraint-free state veterans' facility, is that other residents have difficulty with demented residents anywhere around them. Alert residents constantly complain to the nurses to 'get them (persons with memory loss) back to the wacky ward,' and harass the demented residents, making them the butt of jokes. Staff tries to protect the demented residents, but this is difficult to do while allowing them maximum freedom to ambulate about the building."

"I wish other residents could gain empathy and understanding of the demented residents' limitations, but that is an impossibility. Nursing staff themselves, from other units, view our demented residents as 'combative, agitated, and violent.' Although my residents with dementia do have these moments, so many times it is due to staff approach, environmental factors (overstimulation), and/or pain and discomfort. I wish all the staff would understand 'demented' is not another term for 'criminally insane.'"

One administrator tells this sad story: *"One summer, three of the residents obtained paint from the arts and crafts department and told some of the Alzheimer's residents they could help the nurses by*

☨

painting the courtyard furniture. The confused residents were so proud of their contribution, and the instigators watched and laughed, waiting to see the nurses' reactions. This is a travesty!"

Financial concerns often prevent adequate training programs and problem awareness issues from getting the attention they deserve:

"Nurses like myself in special care Alzheimer's units are helpless without financial backing, to educate ourselves and our staff, and to educate our governmental agencies about the need to have special care units for Alzheimer's patients. It is up to society to open the eyes of administrators and policy-makers. These are not just policy issues we are dealing with. They are issues that effect the behavior of residents, family, and staff alike. Recent research into the effects of architectural cueing and programs in Alzheimer's special care units demonstrates the real benefits of separating out persons who have Alzheimer's disease from the non-demented elderly in care facilities. It does make a difference. In addition, special training in understanding and caring for an Alzheimer's residents can make a remarkable difference in the quality of life for each person with Alzheimer's disease. How can we combine our efforts to educate our government about these needs?"

Another nurse writes, *"I wish the government would understand that Alzheimer Disease, which steals the mind and breaks the heart, needs far more money for research into the cause of the disease. As our population ages, and the number of people with Alzheimer Disease increases, our health care facilities will be overburdened and so will family caregivers who must provide round-the-clock care for their loved ones with Alzheimer's. The emotional and financial drain is enormous."*

If the government does step in, this nurse fears the repercussions:

"With all the current government hassles, most nursing home personnel are so freaked already about regulations, getting things

done on time, and paperwork, they spend all their time with their noses in residents' charts and barely know the resident himself. Will government interference only add to the dilemma?"

"Surely it would be better to provide research money now and find the causes of Alzheimer's and methods of preventing its onset. It would be cheaper in the long run than providing care and support for those with Alzheimer's," argues another nurse professional.

An additional problem facing staff in nursing homes is expressed this way:

"One of the hardest things in caring for Alzheimer's patients in a nursing home is trying to understand why it takes so long for a doctor to get back to us on urgent matters. I sometimes think they consider our Alzheimer's residents less important just because they won't remember the delay in care. But we caregivers know. And we really resent their lack of caring."

This nurse appeals to the administrators of care facilities:

"I wish more administrators understood the severity of problems facing the staff in care facilities today. Inadequate facilities for Alzheimer's patients often prevent families from seeking long-term care placement of their loved ones. It is a constant battle with no real solutions once the pattern is established. However, I have seen strong, educated administrators take over such situations and turn them around. But it must begin at the top—with the education of the owners and administrators. Without their understanding and support, changes within the facility are impossible."

The Need for Better Education

Numerous health care personnel shared their views on the need for proper education for themselves, the families, and their staff about Alzheimer's disease:

"When I first heard the words 'Alzheimer's disease,' I used to

❡

equate it with 'insanity.' Now knowing more about the disease process, I understand how wrong I was. All caregivers: families, professionals and volunteers, need to be educated more about this disease."

"I try to help our nursing staff understand we are in a very rural area and there aren't many support groups in our area to assist families in dealing with Alzheimer's disease. As a matter of fact, there aren't any support groups within 50 miles of our town. The only support group meets in the morning once a week in a town 50 miles away. Most of our family members are working during this time. So it falls on our nursing staff and administration to help these families, to offer support and understanding, and education. But where do we get our information and the time to learn and share it?"

This nurse agrees with the fact that the responsibility of education falls on the nurses and administrators:

"It is up to us nursing home administrators to offer educational classes for our staff to help them assist families cope with their emotions. I see families turning to doctors to gain the support they need when the diagnosis is Alzheimer's disease. Doctors do not have the time to sit with a family and talk them through their emotions. It's up to us."

One nurse professional lamented the same frustration about understanding her role as caregiver for Alzheimer's patients:

"I know Alzheimer's disease is a progressive brain deterioration. However, it is difficult for us (professionals) to find reliable information about this disease. We need to learn from the experiences of caregivers who have come before us. Then we need to continue to share the information we have learned."

Sharing Insights and Caregiving Ideas

Caring for persons with Alzheimer's disease is both unique and often mysterious. There are no textbooks written for health care professionals which give them the "how-to's" of care. The truth is, most professionals have learned mostly from former or current caregivers. In fact, most never even heard the terminology "Alzheimer's disease" in their training. In the following excerpts, nurses share insights and ideas for better understanding and care:

"It is so important for all caregivers of persons with Alzheimer's disease to be open and understanding in their approach," encourages this nurse. *"This means learning how to assess patients for confusion at the time you are addressing them. Most patients have good days and bad days, meaning they are much more alert on some days than others. This information helped guide my care approach for patients with Alzheimer's disease."*

"I am a professional caregiver for persons with Alzheimer's disease. I wish administrators and other professional caregivers understood that persons with this insidious disease DO NOT understand what is happening to them, and require extreme patience and understanding when being cared for. Therefore, it would be my wish that facilities would have an increased staff for the Special Care Unit and other departments caring specifically for those with dementia."

One family member begs professional caregivers to remember *"that the patient is not just a patient. They belong to families who love them and are looking out for their best interest."*

Another professional caregiver encourages her fellow co-workers with these words:

"I wish that when helping an individual with personal care, caregivers would think about things from the perspective of the person they are helping. I cannot begin to imagine what it must be like to

have someone putting diapers on you, bathing you, etc., all of that in addition to being aware of your own cognitive decline. It is very important to remember you are caring for an ADULT, not a child who doesn't know any better."

"I work to help my patient understand that I am her friend," a nurse assistant remarks. *"I love and respect her. I would never harm her. I will continue to work with her to maintain as much of her independence as possible."*

A wise nursing supervisor instructs her staff this way: *"Many of the family members will want to share with you the life and personality of their loved one with Alzheimer's disease. Listen to them—and learn. You need to ask them questions about the personality of their loved one so you can learn from them. Treat the family with dignity and do not look down on them as 'the survivors.' You need to praise their efforts and remind them of just how important they are to the continuing care of their loved one."*

"I work as an administrator in a nursing home and I see families struggling to understand why their loved one doesn't remember them. These signs of guilt that a family member displays with anger, are sometimes aimed towards the nursing staff and sometimes at other residents or towards their loved one. This is a very devastating disease which affects everyone. I try to explain to the nursing staff that the anger a family member is expressing is more often confusion and guilt on the part of the family."

Another nursing director on an Alzheimer's special care unit teaches a lesson this way:

"Recently one of my aides told a family, 'We need to remember the Alzheimer's disease victim no longer has his personality.' Even though this was her attempt to 'help' the family, this statement is disturbing for two reasons: the word 'victim,' and the statement itself. If this caregiver was trying to explain a change in personality to a

family member in these words, it has no positive value. Experience has taught caregivers that each and every person with Alzheimer's disease has a personality. Yes, it changes and needs to be recognized by family members and staff. Together we learn how to care for persons with Alzheimer's disease and their families."

"Please, caregivers, never call a person who has Alzheimer's disease a 'victim,'" advises another nurse. *"This sets up a negative connotation many family members have a hard time overcoming. In fact, many will only hear the word 'victim,' and will have difficulty moving beyond that. In addition, family members need time to accept the truth of this disease: this loved one will never be the same, and neither will the family. A disease in the brain has changed this person forever."*

One nurse relates this story:

"People with Alzheimer's have a disease which is incurable. The process can be slowed but deterioration will continue. Too many professionals say, 'Why invest time in such a 'lost cause.' I was told this by a intern doing his residency in emergency medicine when I was an emergency room nurse. I told this young doctor that one day he will eat and choke on those words. Three years later, I asked him how many times has he had to eat those words. This doctor said, 'I never knew the majority of our clients are of the senior population and the majority of these have Alzheimer's. I have choked on those words many times during my short time in this profession.'"

"(I feel that the) 'lost cause' theory is very widespread throughout the medical and public realm," continued this ER nurse. *"As for Alzheimer's disease, we know today there is no cure, but education is a very important way to assist with understanding this devastating disease. Education needs to be goal-directed. And it needs to be initiated at the basic educational levels for nurses and doctors."*

X

"The best advice for caregivers is to learn all you can about caring for a person with Alzheimer's disease," advises another health care professional. *"They are different, thus making their care different from the care of all other elderly people. Because of cognitive challenges, persons with Alzheimer's disease cannot interpret real pain, discomfort or illness. Often they act out and are deemed as an 'agitated' patient, when, in fact, they have a bladder infection causing much stress and pain. Try to understand that all behavior is purposeful. It has a message. The competent caregiver will discover the message behind the behavior."*

Another professional caregiver expresses the same idea this way:

"When a patient is unable to speak and make me aware of their pain, it makes my caregiving more complicated. I try my best to anticipate what may be wrong, understanding that this patient with Alzheimer's disease cannot TELL me where it hurts."

This nurse administrator offers her insight on patient care:

"It is most important to show your respect for the confused patient. One good rule of thumb to remember is that often the patient will 'mirror' your own behavior and attitude. It's a reciprocal relationship between the caregiver and the person with Alzheimer's disease. This means if you are impatient and rude, you might expect the same behavior from the person for whom you are caring. So take the time to listen, empathize, and treat with TLC, and you will probably get the patient to cooperate and do whatever it is you need to do."

Regarding cooperation of patients with Alzheimer's disease, one nurse offers this suggestion:

"As a nurse professional, I have been doing memory testing of Alzheimer's patients for the past three years. Sometimes I see the same patient every few weeks for months. Knowing they will never remember me from visit to visit, I always approach them as if it is the very first time we are meeting. I begin with a smile, a kind word

about their appearance, and sometimes a touch on the arm. I introduce myself as a nurse who needs their help on a special study I am doing. Then I ask them if they are willing to help me. I have never had one patient refuse to be interviewed. In fact, they often appear flattered that I would ask for their help. They still need to be needed. They need to feel worth as a human being."

A young professional caregiver speaks out on rights of the person with Alzheimer's disease in these words:

"A person with Alzheimer's disease has the same rights as the rest of us, and they deserve the same respect we give to all individuals. When I first became a professional caregiver, I witnessed something which made me physically sick. A particular resident at the facility had very progressive Alzheimer's disease, and was easily confused. A fellow caregiver knew this, and he would deliberately hide behind furniture, calling out the resident's name, and then laughing at the woman's confused reaction. Of course the caregiver was fired, but I wonder how long this went on before someone spoke up about this atrocity!"

Even volunteers share insights that may assist in the care of the Alzheimer's patients:

"I wish someone would have told me earlier that Alzheimer's disease was what their parent was afflicted with prior to their being institutionalized. Sometimes we volunteers have to go through 'baptism by fire' before we are aware of the disease robbing this person from our understanding of why they may not be reacting normally to situations."

An education coordinator/activities director offered these suggestions:

"At our facility we strive to improve the quality of life for the residents who have Alzheimer's disease. We try to do this three ways: through education, increasing social interaction with a program of

regular visits by volunteers, and by increasing physical exercise of residents which also increases strength and sometimes even awareness. Some of our local councils on aging provide pamphlet guides which help us to aid the visitor/volunteer in activities and social interactions making visits more pleasant and enjoyable."

Promoting the advantages of exercise programs, another facility director proposes:

"At our special care facility, we provide exercise programs which meet the individual functional needs of each client. We integrate strength training with nutrition for maximum quality of life for our frail elderly. Additional methods to improve the quality of life for Alzheimer's residents are animal relationship programs and music therapy, which we are soon planning to incorporate soon."

"Try to anticipate any stress the resident may encounter," encourages this administrator. *"A good caregiver will look for ways to help the Alzheimer's patient relax in situations that knowingly will cause stress."*

To enhance caregiving skills, a nurse assistant offers this suggestion:

"I often think about the loss of the past person, and try to think of what that person was like before he or she got this disease. I think about the dignity lost through the invasion of Alzheimer's disease in the people I care for. It makes my caregiving more meaningful."

"When you meet resistance to care, look beyond the behavior," voices another caregiver. *"To accomplish this, I ask myself: Is the patient tired? Is the patient frustrated? Is he/she afraid of a certain procedure or event? Is he/she particularly confused today? Or, is the patient in pain?"*

"I have an idea to help us get to know each individual resident a little better," says this caregiver. *"Why not have residents wear a bracelet or ID tag with such things as: 'Loves to garden;' 'hates carrots;' 'was an avid dancer;' 'loves animals;' 'loved to cook.'"*

Love and Protection . . . and Dedication

There is no doubt caregivers in nursing homes and assisted living facilities are some of the most dedicated, patient, loving care "givers" in the industry. One devoted caregiver expresses her thoughts this way:

"I wish everyone understood I voluntarily give care to this woman from my heart, and that even though I realize she is incapable of loving, she is very deserving of being loved. I wish people would realize the sacrifices I make and not be frightened by her demented behavior. If more people were less ignorant about the disease, it would make being a caregiver much easier and less stressful for this loved one. It would be so nice if family members took her out for a drive, talked to her on the phone, or even acknowledged she is still alive. I give to her without question, and the rewards I receive are immeasurable."

"The saddest things are actually when the fog lifts and the patient suddenly realizes something is terribly wrong," attests an assisted living facility nurses' aide. *"The behaviors and the realities of Alzheimer's disease are easily dealt with, but when you look into clear eyes and see the person as they used to be, you can't help but grieve for the loss, and feel their pain, and pray that the fog returns so that at least they don't know what's happening to them."*

A retired nurse/volunteer who works in an Alzheimer's unit tells us that the saddest thing for her is *"the inability to really do anything to help."* She continues, *"I just have to stand and watch this person degenerate, and to watch the frustration of families and friends, whom the victim no longer recognizes. I wish someone could have told me earlier that this type of work would be so difficult. I get so attached to not only the residents, but to their families."*

"As a nurse in a long term care facility, I see all kinds of reactions to people with Alzheimer's," comments another caregiver. *"For the past two years, my daughters, ages 11 and 12, have done*

volunteer work at the facility where I work. They look forward to coming to the facility so they can assist with the care of these residents. At times they ask why a certain resident gives a particular reaction to an activity they are doing with them, since such a reaction scares them. I explain that sometimes the resident is not responsible for the reactions she gives and the best way to help this resident is to show you care and love them. This is a lesson well-taught at an early age."

"One of the sweetest memories I have," tenderly recalls a volunteer caregiver, *"is the day I told one of the female residents her dress was beautiful and the colors of trees. It was like she fell in love with her dress, and looked at each print for hours. At dinner time, she spread the skirt of her dress over the table like a fine tablecloth, still admiring its beauty!"*

Another caregiver reflects, *"Once I brought my 80-year-old friend who has Alzheimer's disease to the window so she could view the foliage. It was as if she had seen this for the first time in her life. I cried."*

"When I first heard my friend's mother had Alzheimer's disease, I offered to go regularly to the nursing home with my friend and visit with her mother. I wanted to be there to support my friend. Yet I learned the beauty of unconditional love between mother and daughter," this observer admits.

"Working with Alzheimer's residents is one of the hardest things I've ever done," says another. *"Sometimes my mind drifts apart from caregiving and I try to imagine what they were like when they were young, doing things like shopping and housework. Now they need total care—like an infant. They need all the love you can give them. I love all of them like they were my family. And I feel that they will give you all the love they can."*

"Smile, call the patient by name, tell him how glad you are he is part of your day," suggests this caregiver. *"Engage him in*

❦

conversation. Talk, reminisce, sing. Your body language and your tone of voice carry far more credibility to this confused, frightened patient than the words you are actually saying. And include physical touch. This is a basic need and an important way of communicating care."

"*The most frustrating thing about caring for persons with Alzheimer's disease is watching the heartbreak it causes to families, especially when the victim is a younger person,*" notes one nurse. "*Watching these younger people who have dementia and need to be admitted to a care facility is so sad. They seem to still understand what is happening to them, yet they can't stop it. They need to know they are loved, no matter what,*" a caregiver proclaims.

A nurse defines her feelings in this way:

"*My home unit is an intermediate level unit, and I have been filling in on this special care unit for the last eight months until a supervisor is hired. Never have I enjoyed caring for residents so much. My residents with Alzheimer's disease are very child-like in many ways and respond to nurturing in ways that more oriented residents do not. Although it is heartbreak for families, they are a joy to me.*"

There can be no doubt that caregiving of patients with Alzheimer's disease presents unique challenges. There can also be no doubt that most caregivers in nursing home settings give from the heart. Perhaps their sharings will enlighten readers in their understanding and empathy for the problems and concerns of those who truly care about their patients.

❧

11
RECOGNIZING
BEHAVIOR CHANGES

The very essence of human thinking and reasoning elicits mass confusion when trying to understand the behavior of a person with Alzheimer's disease. In order to understand and better cope with the behavior changes which accompany Alzheimer's disease, one must begin to "join the journey," so to speak, of a person who is experiencing such symptoms. Caregivers have found it necessary to revise their thinking about what may be causing such changes. Blaming the person with Alzheimer's disease, or blaming one's self, only complicates the behavior problem issues. It is imperative to understand that the person with Alzheimer's disease, exhibiting unusual behavior symptoms, is not the same person who was once an independent adult with full thinking capabilities. A person with Alzheimer's disease cannot remember, and he is not aware that he cannot remember.

Individuals with Alzheimer's disease exhibit behaviors which are extremely changeable in nature and vary greatly from day to day. A person with Alzheimer's disease is exhibiting <u>normal</u> behavior for a person with Alzheimer's disease. The best caregiving methods are learned by understanding such behavior through listening, observing and sharing caregiving experiences.

A nurse caregiver offers this advice:

"Some days the patient with Alzheimer's disease may seem almost normal or more normal. But remember their reality is very different from yours. You cannot change THEM; you can only control your own reactions to their behavior."

"What works one day for one patient may not work with another patient," this caregiver notes. *"The same strategy may also not work for the same patient on a different day."*

"Don't sweat the small stuff," simply puts a caregiver/aide. *"You'll stay healthier and cope better with that slant on things."*

An added tool to better understanding is the need to interpret and assess changes in function and behavior in relation to what the behavior is really indicating. Something like agitation may indicate a urinary tract infection and nothing more. Often acting-out behavior is misinterpreted and the real cause, a physical cause, is not discovered until much later. Persons with Alzheimer's disease are not able to express their discomforts, pain or illnesses. Word recall and difficulty with short-term memory compound the problems. It is up to the caregiver to interpret behavior and look to physical causes before jumping to psychological conclusions. Here are some of the more common behavior problems noted in persons with Alzheimer's disease: aggression, bathing resistance, death and grief reactions, delusions and hallucinations, denture problems, depth perception difficulties, driving responsibilities, eating problems, emotional problems, hearing problems, medications, moving, pacing, pain perception, reality disorientation, sleep problems, sundowning, and wandering.

Aggression

One of the greatest concerns of caregivers, both family and professionals, is a person with Alzheimer's disease who becomes aggressive. Their combative behavior, shouted threats, hitting, pounding or throwing things result in fear for the safety of both the caregiver and the person for whom they care. This is often the point at which the family decides this person can no longer be safely cared for at home. Frequently a nursing home is the only alternative. An administrator at a nursing home which cares for persons with Alzheimer's disease has this to say:

"In our nursing home we pay special attention to residents who are aggressive. Emphasis has to be on solving the problem that is causing the aggressiveness, and not on the behavior itself. Nursing homes should have a plan of action for the staff to handle such behavior, and this plan should be readily available for the asking by family members. I encourage families to investigate the plan of action for aggressive behavior before their loved one is placed in a care facility."

Another nursing home administrator explains their special care unit policies in this way:

"At our facility all nursing staff has training in Alzheimer's disease and combative behavior. We have a rule that if a resident is combative, a second aide could assist, but any help beyond that must come from a nurse who would assess the resident. I also use occupational therapists to help the aides handle residents who are combative. They are often able to figure out ways of doing things which are less stressful to the residents and safer for the staff. It is important for families to know what we are doing and how we are following through if you get reports of your loved one having frequent outbursts of aggressive behavior."

A head nurse in a special care unit advises this procedure if a family is getting reports about a loved one's aggressive behavior:

"I would advise you, first of all, to make sure you have 'power of attorney' so you can personally have the right to read the medical records.' Go over the nurses' notes and ask for all of the incident reports generated when there were problems. This will give you a better idea of exactly what happened. You will also want to know if your loved one has had a problem with a particular staff person in the past few months of care, and if so, is your loved one upset or intimidated by this particular staff member. If there is no pattern there, next examine what changes have taken place in the environment: a new room? new roommate? new routine? Also ask to see the care plan. This will give you a clue as to the attention given

this behavior, and whether the plans to remedy the situation are being followed. I also highly advise hiring a case manager who is available as certified personnel, who could visit often and act as an advocate for your loved one with aggressive behavior."

One professional caregiver offers this solution: *"Behavior modification, I believe, is the foremost method for solving aggressive behavior problems. What do I mean by behavior modification? Simply put, it means finding the <u>triggers</u> that cause disturbing behavior and then modifying the <u>environment</u> to change the patient's behavior."*

Behavior modification is becoming the mode of choice for understanding and handling aggressive behavior in those with Alzheimer's disease. The following quote, however, clearly indicates how often "behavior modification" can be misinterpreted by the caregiver:

"The saddest thing may be the idea of behavior modification. How can anyone modify the behavior of someone who suffers from Alzheimer's disease? How tormented are the patients who are being constantly told to remember something they will easily forget!"

The downside of behavior modification is the tremendous time such supervision may expend due to the need to individualize such care. Two staff members share these views:

"The sad reality is that most nursing homes do not consider it cost effective to allow so much staff time to go into individual care when you have so many to care for. Behavior modifications which target triggers of the undesirable behavior, and then a baseline, are far too time consuming from the facility's point of view."

"The truth is that most nursing homes are understaffed and follow the old traditional medical model of care. Mental health needs are at the very bottom of that list."

Families need to ask caregivers for specific information about behavior modification. One caregiver suggests a family member approach the staff with this:

"I understand behavior modification as the act of finding the triggers which cause unacceptable and aggressive behavior, and then modifying the environment to help change the patient's behavior. Do you use behavior modification in this facility? If so, how exactly is that done?"

Bathing Resistance

All too often caregivers find bathtime a real struggle in caring for persons with Alzheimer's disease:

"Bathing is one of the most difficult tasks for the caregiver to accomplish," a nurses aide explains. *"Many Alzheimer's patients have a fear of water. A bath can be scary and confusing for a person who does not fully comprehend what is happening."*

One family caregiver offers this suggestion:

"I try to get everything ready ahead of time, gathering the soap, towel, powder, and lotion into the bathroom, and then saying 'Mom, your bath is ready.' Because, if I would ASK Mom if she wanted to take a bath or WHEN she wanted her bath, her answer was always negative. I think the matter-of-fact directive works best."

Many caregivers have learned that merely trying to remove an individual's clothing and attempting to bathe a resistant person can lead to anger, frustration and aggressive behavior. A person with Alzheimer's disease cannot remember from the time you <u>inform</u> him you are going to bathe him to the actual bathing procedures. Often an individual feels violated and doesn't understand why a <u>stranger</u> is attempting to disrobe and touch him.

"It is always a sad and discouraging day when family caregivers discover their loved one can no longer remember routine tasks," one social worker explains. She continues, *"The very nature of the disease robs this person of remembering the steps in once-familiar tasks. Often the most mundane tasks of daily grooming, bathing, and*

dressing become overwhelming to a person with Alzheimer's disease. We need to share ideas in coping and caring."

This loving husband shares his observation and advice:

"Sometimes I heard my wife crying out to the aides who were trying to bathe her: 'What are you doing to me?' She seemed to be put into an ugly, resistive mood. The aides had forgotten that she does not remember from day to day what is done in routine care, and she must be reminded and reassured of their loving concern for her. She does not remember them or whatever relationship they think they might have established with her previously. They must again and again, with each new encounter, remind her of their loving concern and what they are about to do to her."

Here are some other practical tips about routine grooming tasks which creative caregivers have shared:

"If bathing is a problem, know that the bath does not have to be given daily and may actually be damaging to fragile skin. Daily washing of hands, face and genital area are the only daily essentials."

"I've noticed that each person seems to have a 'best' time of day—this is the time the bath should be given. Also try to give the bath the same time each day—many Alzheimer's patients prefer routine."

"I find that being matter-of-fact is the best approach to bathtime. I say, 'It's time to take your bath now,' instead of 'Would you like to take your bath now?' If the individual needs assistance with cleaning the genital area, I use that same calm and matter-of-fact approach."

"If you organize all the bath items ahead of time and lay them out in use order, it makes the bathing task less confusing for an Alzheimer's patient. Also make certain the bathing area is safe, e.g. rubber mat, grab bars; or consider a shower stool to avoid having to step into a tub."

"Let the individual do as much of the bath as possible, even if it takes reminding of each step of the way. If the individual appears frightened or resistant, distract him or her with compassionate conversation. Also keep in mind that sometimes resistance is due to arthritic pain during bathing, yet the person with Alzheimer's disease is often unable to verbalize such pain."

"I remind my aides never to use bubble bath or bath oils as these can make it slippery for the patient and the staff. In addition these oils may cause urinary tract infections."

"Remember to dry the skin thoroughly and apply lotion as necessary. While drying the skin, this is a good time to be alert to any bruises, skin discoloration or injuries and to treat them appropriately. Many persons with Alzheimer's disease are elderly, with delicate skin, so good skin care can be essential in preventing infections."

The following chapters on "Creative Caregiving" and "Compassionate Communication" will offer additional suggestions for approaches to overcoming resistance to accomplishing routine tasks.

Death and Grief Reactions

Because of memory loss, many persons with Alzheimer's disease often do not remember that a dear relative or friend has passed away, even if the death occurred many years ago. Many are "waiting for" or believe they saw or spoke to a relative that is, in fact, dead. If directly reminded of that loved one's death, they may experience the grief of that passing all over again, as if hearing it for the first time. It is often agonizing for the family to realize their loved one does not even remember the death of their spouse, parent, or child. It is just so difficult to understand how that mind works, and that something so profound as the death of a close family member cannot be remembered.

"My Mom often believes my father and her other deceased relatives are all alive, and she grieves all over again when she learns

they're no longer with us," explains a dedicated daughter. *"At first I played along and pretended I didn't hear her questions about them. But ignoring her inquiries only made it worse. She got very persistent. So now I try validating her feelings, and then I add a distraction. I say something like 'You really loved Dad, didn't you, Mom? Let's go get something to eat now.' Mom's short attention span can be a blessing in disguise because she is so easily distracted."*

An administrator of a nursing care facility gives this advice to her staff:

"Encourage your patient to talk, especially about a deceased relative, remembering the good things, and then lead that conversation into something entirely different. Try something like this: 'Oh, your wife was born in Detroit? I lived in Detroit for a while. Did you go to the movies there?' and so on."

"When Mom starts talking about our deceased family members, I've taught my Dad how to change the subject and divert Mom to another idea," an experienced daughter/caregiver says. *"He is getting good at it and it can save his own peace of mind."*

Another wise young daughter learned to "join the journey" or "play the game" with her aging Mom whose husband had died several years before. When her Mom would forget that her husband had died, and asked "Where is Kevin?" the empathetic daughter would say, *"You really miss him a lot, don't you, Mom. He was so special. He had the greatest smile. I think our Jason has his smile. Guess what Jason did yesterday? He played in his first ball game. . ."* She just continues in another vein, after validating what was said. This daughter did not ignore her mother's thought or question. She learned to validate and distract. This method provides dignity and worth to the patient with Alzheimer's by acknowledging that their thoughts and words are valuable. Caregivers will reap the rewards of continuing conversations, without corrections or denials of what is being said. Respond to the feeling behind the statement, not to the words themselves.

These caregivers have the best answer and use the recommended communication techniques of validation and distraction. It only frustrates a person with Alzheimer's disease more if their comment or question is ignored. So acknowledgment of the statement is an important part of loving communication. However, because those with Alzheimer's disease are easily distracted to another topic or activity, it is best to use that technique to avoid the pain of grief or sadness to erupt anew each time the deceased person is mentioned.

Delusions and/or Hallucinations

Often people with Alzheimer's disease will see and hear things that are not actually there. The paranoia of delusionary thinking may cause exceptional family problems. A loved one may constantly accuse the person he is closest to of stealing or lying or other things. This sometimes go hand-in-hand with hallucinatory behavior. Some even talk to people they believe are in the room with them.

"My mom had conversations with people that I could never see," a caregiver relates with obvious dismay. *"She would tell me we had to be quiet because there were children sleeping in the next room. Often she tells me we need to clean up because her mom and dad, who have been dead for 40 years, are coming to visit!"*

"The saddest thing was when my father became paranoid and was convinced that everyone was after his money. He became withdrawn and hateful," a saddened daughter remarks.

An observant son has this to say about his mother's paranoia:

"She thought the people on the TV were in her house and talking to her. They ruled her life. She was afraid to turn off the television because she didn't want to make them mad. When she left her house she kept the lights and TV on to keep them happy."

Since those with Alzheimer's disease truly live in this present moment, many can no longer distinguish reality from make believe. It is impossible to try to argue or talk them out of it. If there is no danger to themselves or anyone else, professionals agree it is best to go along with their delusions without confrontation and arguing.

Denture Problems

Several professional caregivers and family members wrote about denture problems. A geriatric nurse had this good advice:

"It has been my experience that people with Alzheimer's disease do not do well with <u>new</u> dentures. They cannot remember getting new dentures, so they will think these dentures do not belong to them, spit them out, and often hide them. If they have not worn them for a while, they often are too ill to sit for another refitting, and the cost seems to be an unneeded expense if the person is doing well without dentures. So as loving family members, you are the only ones who can decide if there is a chance your loved one will keep them in, and whether or not you will be able to keep replacing them if they are lost, broken or hidden. Nothing replaces good oral hygiene, of course."

Another caregiver adds:

"When my Mom first came to live with us, in the early stage of her disease, she needed some serious dental work. She got full dentures and did well for several months. But as her Alzheimer's disease progressed, and the dentures became loose due to bone recession, the dentist visits became chaotic and frightening to her. She would not tolerate them. So she went to eating pureed food and the problem was solved—no dentures."

"Seeing our parent deteriorate mentally, grow old physically, and then refuse dentures, seems to add to our burdens as family caregivers," one daughter admits. *"The adjustment to my Mom's 'toothless' look was not an easy one for me. My mother suddenly didn't look quite like my mother, not to mention that she had long ago stopped acting like my mother! But she told me she 'enjoyed' not having to be bothered by her dentures."*

❧

An experienced caregiver shares these words of wisdom:

"Our dentist gave this analogy of why elderly people hide or take out ill-fitting dentures: 'It is like kicking off your shoes which didn't fit well and just going barefoot.' He said they probably felt lots better with no teeth than with the old dentures that had gotten loose and were annoying."

Depth Perception Difficulties

In caring for persons with Alzheimer's disease it is most important to interpret their behavior symptoms with an understanding of their thought processes. Most persons with Alzheimer's disease experience a problem with depth perception at times. This will result in sometimes resistant, or what may be perceived as abnormal, behavior.

A nurse in a care facility offers this helpful observation:

"I have seen persons with Alzheimer's walking from a sidewalk onto the grass and stopping to 'test' the terrain with one foot before proceeding forward. They just cannot properly 'process' the change from the cement to the grass. They see it clearly, but the brain does not process it, and this causes fear of the unknown territory to a person with Alzheimer's disease."

One nurse tells this story about the procedure of having a person with Alzheimer's disease stand on a scale for simple weighing, and it turning into a resistant and time-consuming task:

"The patient would balk at being encouraged to stand on the scale, until I discovered the reason for this: the scale had a black base. For a person with Alzheimer's disease who is experiencing difficulty in thought processes , the black base looked like a HOLE. The brain was warning the patient this might be a HOLE into which she or he could fall. Once the color of the scale base was changed to white, the fear of stepping up on the scale diminished!"

It becomes increasingly clear that caregivers must go OUTSIDE of their own realm of reality and try their best to assess the patient's reason for adverse behavior. If you are fortunate enough to discover a piece of the understanding "puzzle," do share that information with others.

Driving Responsibilities

The issue about the elderly driving is a very delicate one, especially when it comes to Alzheimer's disease. With this disease affecting some people as young as 40, Alzheimer's patients who drive become a major safety issue. Should people who are diagnosed with Alzheimer's disease have their licenses revoked or suspended? *"Not necessarily,"* say memory disorder specialists. *"Since Alzheimer's disease affects different people differently, the driving issue has to be answered on an individual basis. The family and physician must look at the person with Alzheimer's disease and determine how the disease has affected his or her normal functioning and reactions. Driving tests should include some basic neurological testing to see if the person can follow simple commands such as 'turn left here,' or 'stop' at this particular place."*

A family member responds:

"My father who has Alzheimer's disease was reluctant to listen to me or Mom regarding his safety (and the safety of others) in driving. But he did listen to his doctor when he said it was time to turn over his keys."

The most serious issue, of course, is that of safety. For the person with Alzheimer's disease who still retains many cognitive functions and the fight to remain independent, driving is a source of many arguments. In a recent statement the American Psychiatric Association recommended that doctors should order Alzheimer's patients to give up their car keys because *"victims can cause car crashes even in the early stages of the mind-robbing disease."* The Association further advises physicians to write a prescription against driving *"so that relatives have something to use as leverage when patients forget."* In some cases, doctors might have to consider breaching patient confidentiality to report dangerous Alzheimer's drivers to state authorities.

One wise caregiver/wife offers this advice:

"When my husband went for his license renewal, I called ahead and asked the Bureau to revoke his license for the safety of all concerned. Even though he knew his judgment and memory were impaired, he never wanted to give up his license. It caused many arguments between us and no amount of reasoning on my part made any difference. I hated to go behind his back, but I felt this was a life and death issue. The State was very cooperative."

Eating Problems

Changes in behavior during meals is one area in which several caregivers shared their frustrations. Often families view the behavior of the person with Alzheimer's disease as unacceptable and, frequently, unbelievable. Poor table manners, reluctance to eat, and sheer confusion on the part of the individual with Alzheimer's causes interrupted meals and hard feelings.

"My once 'prim-and-proper' mother was now dumping food on her plate, dripping food from her mouth as she spoke, and sometimes acted like she didn't remember what a fork was for!" this disappointed daughter complains. *"The children would laugh, and I would cry in frustration."*

Having the loved one eat first without distraction, simplifying the task of eating, and ignoring the behavior as much as humanly possible is how more experienced caregivers learn to cope with eating problems. One caregiver found this solution:

"I try giving him only ONE food item at a time on his plate, with only one implement to eat with. This really helps to avoid the confusion of too many things in front of him at once, which would lead to inappropriate behavior and table manners."

Another offers this:

"My father always had impeccable manners at the table. Now we have to practically scold him for taking all the food that is passed and putting it onto his own plate. One way we found to solve this problem is to fill the plates in the kitchen."

"Joining the journey" or "going with the flow" is how many caregivers learn to cope:

"My husband does some strange things with his food now. He puts a pat of butter in his coffee and then tears up bread and puts it in the cup. Then he eats the whole thing with his spoon. What do I do? I just call it his 'coffee soup' and go on."

Another caregiver adds:

"My approach is to not worry about the things that are harmless. I try to keep the environment as safe as possible and just cope with things as they come up. I will never be able to predict what will come next anyway, so there's no way to prepare for it."

Emotional Problems/Feelings

"If there is one thing of which I am certain, it is this: persons with Alzheimer's disease never lose feelings. They know when they feel good or badly about something. They often 'mirror' their caregiver's feelings. They just aren't able to express what they are feeling," a family caregiver says with conviction.

Although persons with Alzheimer's disease most often cannot identify or express their feelings, and in some cases cannot communicate at all, their body language reveals the feelings they are sensing. In addition, a persons with Alzheimer's, more often than not, <u>mirrors</u> the feelings of the person caring for them. *"They are very perceptive, even if they cannot tell you what they are feeling,* a nurse comments. *"Often they can no longer verbally describe feelings of pain, discomfort, fright, or anxiety in words, but their body language tells another story."*

☥

"I hear people say that Alzheimer's people lose their humanity." This caregiver goes on to refute this belief, *"A lot is lost, but not that. Just last week I went to see my mother, and she was sitting next to a woman who's completely nonverbal—a very strange woman. My mother, who has never been that demonstrative, was holding this woman's hand and stroking her face. And I thought: How dare anyone say these people have lost their humanity!"*

A caregiver in a special care unit tells this story to validate how persons with Alzheimer's disease have feelings:

"A rather verbal resident of a special care unit, who scores under 5 points on a 30-point MMSE because she can no longer coordinate her speech with her mind, came into the room of another resident who was very ill and dying. She just sat by the bedside for an hour, and stroked the ill resident's arm. Then, in a fully cognizant moment, she said, 'I don't think she is going to be with us much longer.' What insight! What recognition! So please, don't ever underestimate what might be going on in the mind of a person with Alzheimer's. Often their hearts and heads are fully aware, even if their words or actions do not match."

The following chapters on Creative Caregiving and Compassionate Communication will demonstrate additional points on the emotional feelings of persons with Alzheimer's disease.

Hearing Problems

Unfortunately hearing problems can place an added burden on those persons who are already confused with the verbal word and its meaning. This advice from a nurse-caregiver deserves attention:

"Women's voices are harder to hear than men's voices because of the pitch. Always make a conscious effort to lower the pitch of your voice if you are a female speaking to a person who is hard of hearing. If you know which side of the head the person hears from the best,

talk to that side. Speak slowly and clearly, in short sentences. If the person is wearing a hearing aid, make sure it has batteries. Also make certain that the batteries work, that the hearing aid is turned on, and that the hearing aid is clean and free from ear wax. This seems like such minor instructions, yet for a person with Alzheimer's disease, who also has a hearing problem, words can be doubly confusing. Try to eliminate the problem of hearing so that you can be certain you are only dealing with the memory or dementia problem."

Using Medications for Behavior Problems

Family and professional caregivers shared their views on the pros and cons of using behavior-altering medications to treat persons with Alzheimer's disease:

"Medication should not be the first answer for behavior problems in persons with Alzheimer's disease," a head nurse remarks. *"It may be necessary at some time, but as a director of a special care Alzheimer's unit, it is my experience that once having established an appropriate program for each resident, medication becomes almost irrelevant. I have found an appropriate individualized care program is far more powerful and effective than a drug program."*

"But the burden of this disease is so overwhelming," adds another health care professional, *"that often one-on-one family caregivers have to resort to medicating their loved ones, so they can get some sleep. It's a sad fact, but true."*

As always, it is important to remind caregivers that each person responds differently to drug therapy and other measures. Drugs must be prescribed with caution for those with Alzheimer's disease. Another health care professional offers this advice:

"It is best to start on a low dose, observe closely for side effects, and to frequently reassess with the family and professional team, the benefits versus the risks."

"The extent of over-medicating elderly persons, especially those with Alzheimer's disease, horrifies me," cautions a nurse care provider. *"I see it as a widespread and severely damaging problem."*

A family caregiver questions this reply to her recent inquiry:

"My Mom was sleepy all the time, so I asked the Doctor if we could try to reduce her medications. He said no, because she was docile and not creating any problems in the nursing home. Is that a reason to not reduce her medications?"

A nursing home administrator agrees, *"If we just drugged up all our residents, then no one would cause any problems or hassles all day, because they would all be sleeping in their wheel chairs. This is what some homes feel is the correct solution to behavior problems. Such a sad scenario!"*

"I had difficulty differentiating between changed behavior due to the progression of the Alzheimer's disease or possible side effects of the current medications," another family member remarks. *"How does the doctor determine that psychotropic drugs may become unnecessary as the disease progresses?"*

"I am concerned about how often nursing homes seem to use medications as an answer to behavior problems," voices this nurse-caregiver. *"My professional opinion is that the less psychotropic medications we can use for Alzheimer's patients, the better their quality of life."*

Still another professional encourages all caregivers to *"take a few minutes to read, learn all you can, and talk to other caregivers at support group meetings to explore other alternatives to reduce behavior problems before resorting to drugs to change a behavior."*

"We use hugs and smiles in place of psychotropic drugs—and it works!" enthusiastically says a care facility nurse. *"We've had many new admittances come to our facility on some pretty hefty drugs. I understand that each person is different, but we take the chance of*

occasional aggressive behavior, in favor of showing each resident how much we value him or her as a person. We take pride in the fact that even some of the most aggressive residents melt with the love and affection shown. There are so many variables with this disease. But I am certain that our hugs and love provide the comfort and 'psychotropic' behavior-altering means to combat unacceptable behavior in the majority of cases."

Moving

Any change in location can be overwhelming to a person with Alzheimer's disease. Often moving to a new home, or traveling to even familiar places, triggers added confusion, disorientation, and fear in persons with Alzheimer's disease. These symptoms are exhibited by acting out or arguing. It is also frightening to the caregiver who has difficulty understanding the confusion.

Several caregivers quoted in previous chapters spoke out about the difficulties and behavior changes when a loved one traveled or moved to a new location. Many times these were the first signs of the disease process. However, even in the later stages, a move from a family home to a care center can elicit new behavior problems. The best remedy is love, understanding, and reassuring the person with Alzheimer's disease that they are safe and cared for.

This daughter tells what happened when her Mom moved into the daughter's home:

"Moving Mom into our home seems to have triggered a lot of memories for my Mom. Now she thinks she's a wife and mother, running a household and caring for her children. She believes I am 12, literally, and laughs when I tell her I'm 39 years old."

"Mom was so agitated and paced endlessly when we first brought her to the care center to live," relates another daughter. *"The fright in her eyes devastated me. But a caring staff, and the*

understanding words of their family support group, brought all of us through a difficult situation. Mom seems at peace in her new home now. But it was a long haul—especially for me."

It is not unusual to find families having a more difficult time than the patients in accepting the new situation.

Pacing

Pacing the floor is one of the more common activities of persons with Alzheimer's disease. For some people, pacing seems to be triggered by certain circumstances like a noisy or confusing environment. For others, pacing is just part of their everyday behavior and is related to changes in the brain. *"Always try to assess the reason for the pacing, and eliminate the reason if at all possible,"* suggests a nurse/director.

Some of the triggers which may cause or increase pacing are:
- a change in the environment
- boredom
- emotional reactions such as anger, fear, confusion, anxiety or frustration
- the need for exercise
- constipation
- pain or discomfort
- too much sleep
- hunger or thirst
- the need to use the bathroom

It is a wise and empathetic caregiver who knows her duty well, who will seek to discover the reason for the pacing.

"Even the presence of a maintenance repair man can cause confusion and agitation for my residents, and I notice an increase in pacing," notes one nurse.

"I noticed that my husband didn't seem to be getting enough

exercise and began to pace the floors," remarks a spouse/caregiver, *"so I got a second exercise bike for my husband and now he 'rides' with me when I am exercising. This has been beneficial in helping to reduce his need to wander and pace, not to mention the good of exercising for me."*

However, if pacing is related to changes in the brain, it is unavoidable. If pacing is unavoidable, be aware of these safety precautions:

- set up a secure area in which they can pace without danger of tripping or getting lost
- make certain the individual has supportive, non-slip shoes
- observe feet and legs for swelling, blisters, and redness and treat accordingly
- see that the person is dressed in loose, comfortable clothing
- encourage frequent rest periods by distracting the pacing person to a chair and conversing with that person
- offer frequent snacks to avoid weight loss due to caloric burnout.

Pain Perception

According to a recent (September/October, 1996) article in *Geriatric Nursing Magazine*, pain is very prevalent among the elderly. Authors indicate as many as 85% of the elderly who live in long-term care settings may be experiencing pain, especially from old fracture sites and/ or old surgical sites. Contrary to the belief that persons with Alzheimer's disease cannot <u>identify</u> pain, many try to verbalize their <u>feelings</u> of pain. Those who are unable to recognize or verbalize their pain may exhibit angry outbursts, depression or agitation, or by being totally unable to concentrate, since, in fact, their mind is concentrating on the pain.

A nurse offers this recommendation:

"The person with Alzheimer's needs to be made as comfortable as possible. Any physical problems, no matter how small, adds to the

confusion. Problems like fluid retention and indigestion shouldn't be allowed to go on."

Caring caregivers would never deliberately ignore the pain of a person for whom they were responsible. But how many are actually looking at a frustrating behavior problem as a possible expression of pain for that individual?

"Many persons with Alzheimer's disease can adequately reveal their source of pain. 'Listen' to them through your acute observations," encourages a nurse/caregiver.

Reality Distortion

In referring to a person's digression from reality, one caregiver said this:

"It dawned on me I must be out of my mind to insist on reality."

With this realization, Deborah Hoffman had finally came to terms with the understanding of her elderly mother who was diagnosed with Alzheimer's disease. Deborah's Oscar-nominated video documentary entitled "Complaints of a Dutiful Daughter" gives hope and humor to those who are caring for a loved one diagnosed with Alzheimer's disease. Deborah said that she read and viewed everything she could get her hands on about Alzheimer's disease when she first got her mother's diagnosis. She found the information so depressing and tragic, and she wanted to let caregivers know there was another side of caregiving, a way to cope which was *"bearable."*

Deborah's lesson was to meet her mom *"right where she is at,"* she explained. Deborah taught others how to refrain from insistence of reality, and "play the game," so to speak, to keep the conversation and peace with someone who has Alzheimer's disease. If her mom said it was Tuesday, and in fact it was Sunday, what harm did it do to agree it was Tuesday. Experienced caregivers such as Deborah have provided others with insights and tools which make caregiving not only bearable, but a joy.

Along with reality comes the issue of forgetfulness. Such memory loss, especially of the most current events, are difficult for some caregivers to understand.

"Think of all memories as being written on one piece of paper," suggests one counselor. *"Pretend the long-ago memories or your first childhood memories are at one end of the paper, and your most recent memories (e.g. eating lunch, orientation to time or place) are at the far end. Picture the disease called Alzheimer's destroying brain cells which control memory, but understand that this disease seems to start at the most recent memory end. Start rolling that piece of paper at the short-term end. You can see that many long-ago memories can remain for a long time. Yet the most recent events become 'lost' in the brain, as the paper is rolled."*

Sexual Incidents

Often persons with Alzheimer's disease retain loving feelings, and their need for intimacy and love remain intact far into the progression of their disease. Brain damage due to the Alzheimer's may even heighten the need for sexual activity and decrease sexual inhibitions. Understanding this need may assist caregivers, especially spouses, in their response to the demands of a loved one with Alzheimer's. Many spouses continue to rely on touching, caressing, and nonverbal relations as substitutes for the sex act.

Occasionally in care facilities, persons with Alzheimer's disease relate these needs to one another and seek such intimacy with another resident. Most staff are educated in their appropriate responses. One such administrator advises this approach:

"The key to reaction to sexual incidents is to distract and relocate the persons involved in the sexual circumstance, maintaining your composure and their dignity at the same time. The important ingredient is to help maintain one's dignity. If I find an Alzheimer's

resident engaging in a sexual act, I distract them with something like this: 'Carolyn, I've been looking all over for you. I need you to . . .,' and then lead them away from the area."

Sleep

Most professionals agree, unless there is some physical reason for needing more sleep, older people need no more than eight hours or less sleep per day. One family caregiver shares this idea:

"I've found if I keep Mom active during the day, allow only an hour of napping throughout the day, and don't let her go to bed before nine or ten o'clock, she has much better nights of sleep."

Another daughter relayed this information:

"I tried putting my Dad in day care three days a week and found it increased his social stimulation and activities and allowed for him to actually be tired and sleep better at night."

Some physicians encourage a mild sleep agent to enhance a restful night. One physician tells us:

"We have had particular success using Trazodone to improve sleep and decrease agitation in Alzheimer's disease sufferers. Trazodone is often better tolerated than other drugs. All drugs can cause side effects, and Trazodone is no exception, with postural hypotension and ankle swelling as the main ones I've encountered."

Many caregivers report difficulties with sleep patterns in their loved ones with Alzheimer's disease. This can be so disruptive for the patient, as well as causing sleeplessness for the caregiver. One caregiver describes his difficult situation:

"Sometimes I wish I could crawl into a hole and put it in after me! We have been suffering from sleep problems for months. My wife generally goes to bed around 10 pm without any problem She goes to sleep almost instantly. However, after about three hours, she wakes up disoriented, confused and upset. She wanders around the house,

complaining about the dark, losing something, or even calling for her mother who died 10 years ago. I can get her back into bed, but she repeats the pattern of wandering about every 20 minutes for the rest of the night. A psychiatrist prescribed Perphenazine to control the problem. Initially it helped, but then, as the dosage was adjusted, she became nothing more than a vegetable, sleeping all the time. This was not acceptable and we discontinued the drug. Since then, sleep is becoming more and more rare and precious."

This is precisely why caregivers often need respite, relief from caregiving, to catch up on much-needed sleep. Sleep deprivation can make one feel less energetic and much less tolerant and patient, the very ingredients needed for caregiver survival.

Often mid-day naps for a person with Alzheimer's disease can bring about confusion as to date and time. A short, one-hour nap may confuse some people into believing it is the next day. *"One Saturday night my husband came into the living room all dressed and ready for church following his after-dinner short nap,"* explained this spouse. *"He couldn't realize that it was Saturday night and not Sunday morning. This seems to happen when he wakes up and has a lapse of time concept. Another time he took a nap on a Sunday afternoon, and awakened to go to his Monday doctor appointment, thinking it was Monday. It takes a tremendous amount of coaching and explaining on my part to convince him of the real time and date. It's exhausting!"*

Sundowning

Unique to individuals with acute or chronic confusion such as with Alzheimer's disease is a term called "sundowning" where one becomes more confused, restless and insecure late in the day and especially after dark. Some researchers have attributed this to the fact that the person did not get enough exercise or stimulation during the day, creating a restless feeling at the evening time. Others say it is due to being tired and worn out and in need of sleep, but fighting the need by wandering.

"We can almost see the same correlation in toddlers who have not had a nap," says one researcher. *"They get tired and irritable, but don't know that they need sleep."*

Still other researchers are examining more natural stimulants such as coffee or ice cream (sugar increases hyperactivity in some) which may cause the restless, irritable behavior as the day progresses. The truth is, the jury is still out on this one. Like so many of the behaviors common to those with Alzheimer's disease, more research and understanding is needed. For unknown reasons, an increase in confusion in the late afternoon or early evening, sometimes coupled with restlessness, is common in those with Alzheimer's disease. Some caregivers offered these suggestions:

"I encourage a nap or quiet time with soft music after lunch. This seems to soothe the confused state and keep her calmer as the day wears on."

"I found that it was the ice cream treat I was giving Dad in the late afternoon that was causing a sugar-high like anxiety later in the day."

"Caregivers might also consider decreasing their expectations and demands of the person with Alzheimer's disease during this time of the day. Also check the lighting in your home or facility. Good lighting sometimes can deter confusion. In addition, try orienting the person by telling them the time of the day, where they are, or something that is going on. Perhaps the dark brings fear and confusion."

"Our staff takes turns walking outside with residents. This exercise routine seems to eliminate some of the sundowning effects."

Wandering

Many individuals with Alzheimer's disease seem to cope with their dementia by wandering. Wandering can be extremely dangerous because most Alzheimer's victims do not realize when they are lost. Wandering is one of the main reasons for caregiver burnout—having a loved one who wanders constantly requires 24-hour a day supervision.

One caregiver shares this information:

"Our local Alzheimer's Association works with the local police department through a program known as the Wanderer's Identification Program. This program allows for quick identity of individuals with Alzheimer's who wander. The person with Alzheimer's carries some form of identification, such as a necklace, bracelet or card containing pertinent information: name, address, phone numbers, and the fact that this person is memory-impaired. This type of identification can prevent long hours of confusion and terror for your loved one, and can give peace of mind to you the caregiver. The sooner a lost loved one can be identified, and the families notified, the sooner they can be returned safely to their families."

"I am very lucky because my Mother does not wander or run off like some do. It is one of the scariest things to not know where your parent is, or what is happening to him or her. You know they can't remember to tell anyone where they live. To avoid this problem, my son and daughter-in-law bought Mother an ID bracelet for Christmas one year, and it has my name and phone number the back of it. This is very helpful, but you must remember to put it on in a way that they can't take it off."

Often family members want to keep the "secret" of the Alzheimer's diseased family member to themselves. However one daughter advises, *"Let your neighbors know about your relative's illness so they will understand and offer to help if needed."*

In addition to wearing an ID bracelet, and letting your neighbors know about the disease, notifying the local police of your loved one's condition is also a good idea. Should your family member wander off, you may avoid unneeded worry and concern if you pre-arrange his/ her return.

"I swallowed my pride and alerted my neighbors about my wife's condition," remarks this spouse. *"They have been a God-sent by calling me if they see my wife wandering out of our yard."*

It is also recommended that you use "child-safe" doorknob covers that fit loosely over the door knobs so that only the cover turns, and not the knob itself. New door latches may be indicated, or bells or alarms on opened doors might help prevent an accidental wandering. Some caregivers have even camouflaged the exit doors with a curtain. However, many wander because they need the exercise. At first, allow your loved one to wander outside under your watchful eye, and see if they develop a pattern for their wandering. Then determine if it is a consistent routine that could be incorporated into daily walks. You may find that making provisions for a routine walk may help the individual control wandering at inappropriate times.

Several caregivers shared the horrors of the wanderings of their loved ones, compounded with uncooperative, and often ignorant, law enforcement agencies who offered no assistance:

"Both my mother and father had Alzheimer's disease and were wanderers," laments a former caregiver. *"I had many tragic experiences with a police department which would scold me for not looking after my parents. My Dad got lost while he was walking two times before we took action to prevent his leaving my apartment. The most hurtful thing was the callous attitude of the police when we would phone in a panic to report a missing person. The second time they had actually put him into jail! Why don't they get some training about the proper care and attitude for those wanderers with Alzheimer's disease. We are doing the best we can under the circumstances!"*

"I wish my community would understand that persons with Alzheimer's disease who are discovered as missing must be considered lost, and must be responded to as an emergency," voices another caregiver.

Still another caregiver shares this tragic story:

"My mother wandered away from our home five years ago—and is still 'missing.' Knowing that 60-70 percent of Alzheimer's victims wander, we need to have more vigorous resources for locating missing persons who are memory impaired. For five long years I have been through the guilt and emotional trauma of not knowing where my mother is—or was. I am emotionally drained. Yet I am somewhat comforted with the fact that most people who wander and get lost are returned home safely. However, individuals with Alzheimer's disease DO wander from supposedly secured facilities and homes. Please do everything you can to prevent a tragedy like the one I continue to live with."

Behavior management

All behavior must speak a message for caregivers from the person with Alzheimer's disease. If adverse behavior becomes threatening or dangerous, first try to get the person to stop the undesirable behavior. At the same time, ask yourself if a physical illness or drug reaction might be causing the behavior. Assess the vision and hearing of the person, and/or if something might be upsetting him or her. Keep in mind that persons with Alzheimer's disease are most often unaware of their problem, so they cannot make sense of what is going on. Look for a way in which the behavior can continue in a safe, nondestructive way. Then take the time to reassure the patient that things are all right and that you still care for him or her.

"Sometimes putting your arm around them or giving them a hug is all that is needed to discontinue the unacceptable behavior," one nurse remarks. *"In fact, I think this show of loving concern*

reassures myself as well. I have a very demanding job as caregiver, and I use this technique to rechannel my patients' focus."

"After I handle an adverse-behavior situation, I see if I can get away for a few moments to sort of review what happened, how I managed it, and what I learned from the experience. Sharing the management of difficult behavior can help all the staff, and so I try to do just that," this head nurse comments.

Conclusion

Caregivers could write volumes on the changes in behavior which add interest and astonishment, fear and disappointment to their day— every day. The most important thing to learn is that you will never be able to predict what each new day will bring, and if the behavior is not harmful to a patient or another person, just let it be. If the behavior has the potential to be harmful, try to distract the individual with loving care and reassurance. Then reassess your own attitudes and caregiving actions, and share your responses with others. If at all possible, see the humor in the situation to aid in attitude adjustment and coping skills, and share the humor with other caregivers.

12
CREATIVE CAREGIVING

Caregivers often grow weary with guilt as they question their abilities and care techniques. "Am I doing it right? Am I doing what is best for this person with Alzheimer's disease?" are frequently the questions they ask themselves. "I'm not certain about what to say or do in caring for this person," they admit openly. Why do caregivers believe they should be able to <u>know</u> how to deal with the situations that are occurring? Even professionals offer their best "guesses" for care, based on their knowledge of the disease and experience in caregiving. It is actually the day-to-day caregivers, family and professionals alike, who share their experiences and teach the most about care.

One such experienced caregiver offers this insight:

"Each person with Alzheimer's disease is different and unique. No two persons will follow the exact same path of digression the same way. Thus no two persons will react the same to a given situation. As common as this disease is becoming, experts are a long way off from knowing or understanding the implications of care. Sharing our creative ideas with other caregivers, and being open to trying new approaches suggested by others, are our best tools in developing sound techniques of care."

It is apparent it is not "the experts" who are the teachers of care, but the "experienced" who have taught caregivers the most. Being creative in the caregiving of a person with Alzheimer's disease involves listening, observing, learning new approaches, and most important, sharing ideas with others. Such creative caregiving will lead to more confidence for a caregiver.

"The best thing we can do is to learn how to be flexible in our caregiving and to learn all we can from other people who take care of

those with Alzheimer's disease," rationalizes this caregiver.

"In sharing ideas, we learn new ways to respond to persons who have Alzheimer's disease with compassion and caring and understanding," this caregiver remarks.

Another caregiver agrees, *"I have learned from other caregivers that it is essential to 'go with the flow' —with patience, understanding, cheerfulness, reassurance and HUMOR—always and all ways! There's no other way."*

"If you are going to excel at caregiving, don't stop learning or sharing new ways of caring for the Alzheimer's person," comments a professional caregiver. *"We have all learned from each other—and we keep learning new, creative ways to cope with each individual, each day, in each new experience."*

Following are excerpts from caregiver experiences in an effort to share ideas and insights that may lead to creative, more confident caregiving. They are divided into topics of: activities, day stay programs, pets, music, outings, spirituality, and visiting.

Activities

An array of activities is so important to the creative caregiving of any person with Alzheimer's disease. The truth is, most who have Alzheimer's disease are otherwise healthy and need activities and exercise to preserve good physical maintenance. Memory loss does not necessarily mean one has to give up once-enjoyed activities. It is important, however, not to judge a person's abilities until a new activity is tried and monitored for several days.

There are many new activities which can be tried as long as they do not overwhelm or tax the abilities of one with Alzheimer's. If a particular activity causes frustration or behavior outbursts, discontinue it. The uniqueness of activities with Alzheimer's patients is this: most will not remember the activity from the previous time, so each activity can be like a whole new experience to that person.

"Everyone is different and what works for one person will not necessarily work for another, so a lot is trial and error," notes one activities director. *"Begin with familiar tasks or old hobbies, but if you find it too frustrating because one is aware of one's inability to perform, drop this activity and try it at another time."*

"Provide activities which focus on enjoyment, not achievement," advises another staff member.

"Do remember that most people with Alzheimer's disease cannot initiate an activity," this director reminds us. *" In addition, most will not recall having just done an activity or heard an instruction. So be patient and tolerant."*

"Each new activity has to be tested and monitored for each patient, each *time it is attempted,"* explains a social worker. *"People with Alzheimer's disease change from day to day. Some days they are more alert and capable than others."*

A wise activities director shares this insight:

"Tap into their personalities. If they were very social individuals, they may still enjoy being out around people even if they can't engage in conversation any longer. If they enjoyed more solitary activities, then doing home activities may be best. This is not to say that people don't change. It's just a general rule we have found that works more often than not."

"When a person is in the early to mid-stages of Alzheimer's disease, why does it seem that no one asks the person what they would like to do?" questions an activities therapist. *"I know they may quickly forget the conversation, but many could provide us valuable information about their activity needs if we tried including them more often in the decisions."*

Another caregiver offers this suggestion:

"Take an old hobby and simplify the steps, repeating just one step at a time."

"If someone was never a crafts-type person, it will not be their natural inclination to sit down and fiddle with paper and glue and feel comfortable," remarks an activities coordinator.

Several caregivers took the time to share these ideas for activities:

"Try an old jewelry box full of costume jewelry or an old purse with some of your junk mail in it along with some combs, unbreakable mirror, tissues, keys, and children's play things like a lipstick which has no real color. You can find old costume jewelry at thrift shops and flea markets. Women love to go through it and try different things on."

"Get a bird feeder and place it in a window so the residents can watch."

"Read, look at pictures, listen to tapes. Music is also a great activity for everyone."

"Physical activity is important: taking a walk, tossing a ball, batting balloons."

"Our special care Alzheimer's unit has a great 'walking' plan. Realizing how important it is for our residents to exercise, and, taking advantage of our year-round nice Florida weather, all staff has an opportunity to take residents for a walk during their breaks and/or lunch period. Each time they do so, their name goes into a special drawing for a new, expensive pair of sneakers which is awarded to one lucky 'walker' each month. From directors to volunteer staff, you never saw so many enthusiastic 'walkers,' not to mention satisfied, happy, 'exercised' residents! It benefits everyone!"

The staff at one nursing home, after losing their full-time Activities Director, came up with a unique way to share their time and talent, and at the same time, get to know the residents better:

"We are each requested to give one hour a week of our time and talent sharing an activity in the special care Alzheimer's unit. I play the piano, another staff member reads to the residents, some

teach a craft or skill, and others just toss the ball. Each gives of themselves and we all benefit."

"Make sure your loved one is in a facility which caters to his or her needs," cautions one family member. *"One of the saddest events was when I found my uncle who resided in the Alzheimer's unit of his nursing home, sitting in a pitch black room with a large group of other residents. They had been watching a video movie. The movie had ended and someone had come in and turned off the TV. No one turned on the lights or opened the shades. The residents had just been left sitting in rows in a large dark room. Most were restrained in wheelchairs."*

Day Stay Programs

One rather new approach to activities for adults with dementia and/or Alzheimer's disease is the adult day stay programs. These programs were established to provide two important functions: 1) socialization and appropriate activities for a person with dementia; 2) respite, a break for the caregiver. Studies have shown those in day care regularly seem to plateau for longer periods of time, have less depression, remain cognizant longer, and enjoy the activities.

"Don't wait until you are in a crisis situation to try adult day care," cautions a caregiver/spouse. *"I did. But after a few weeks, I wondered why I hadn't tried this much sooner. My husband is happy and I get to have some time for my self to visit a library, read, and get away from the stress of constant caregiving for a while."*

How do you get a resistant loved one to try a day stay program? Caregivers share these suggestions:

"The key is to find the 'trigger' for your loved one and use that trigger to initiate day stay. What do I mean by that? If your mom did volunteer work in her past, tell her that 'The Club' (your new word for the day stay program) in town is requesting 'helpers' in their program

with the elderly. Ask her if she would 'volunteer' to help the 'older people' by passing out cookies or chatting with the members. Most people, if they think they are contributing to the well-being of others, will gladly 'volunteer' to do so. Then be sure to work out the details with the directors of the program. Most times they are delighted to reinforce your plan."

"We have one former physician with Alzheimer's disease coming to our day stay program to 'make rounds,' and a former teacher coming to 'teach,' a former musician coming to 'entertain the elderly at the club' and even a former dancer who comes to 'teach' others how to dance. Some even go to play cards or just to visit, because it is their 'club,' and that alone gives them a precious reason for attending."

"Our day stay program calls itself 'The Board Room.' We invite the 'board members,' who often come dressed in their suits, to attend a 'meeting,' which in reality is a day stay program for former executives who now have Alzheimer's disease. Each has a purpose (whether real or imagined) in attending because the part of their brain that can remember, remembers only their valuable place at board meetings."

Just think how that feeling would differ from telling your loved one with Alzheimer's disease that they "need to go to day care so you will be watched while I get some time to myself." Instead the "tune" changes when one can say, "The Club just called and they need you to come down today to teach the members how to do the polka." Of course, each day is a new beginning and a new "reminder" of how their services are needed, but that's a small price to pay for a contented and "giving" feeling which accompanies this creative strategy.

Dogs As Protectors/ Pets

A recent newscaster announced the intents of some Humane Societies to initiate the training of dogs for Alzheimer's victims' protection.

These dogs are not trained to be pets, but rather to assist in the care and protection of a person with Alzheimer's disease. They are trained to notify the caregiver by barking and seeking help (or awakening) if their charge awakens, wanders, or is in trouble. The particular couple they featured was a female spouse with crippling arthritis who was wheelchair-bound and could not always quickly get to her husband, who had Alzheimer's disease. The trained dog could alert the spouse/caregiver of any changes in the activities of her patient in another room.

In addition, several nursing homes now allow dogs and cats to live-in and wander freely throughout the facility. They are cared for by staff and loved by the residents. Some bring in puppies who grow up around the residents and remain with them faithfully for many years. Some adopt former greyhound racing dogs who turn out to be compassionate, caring pets for the residents. A recent newspaper article cited the story of a greyhound who just naturally snuggles next to any resident who is crying. It is a great diversion from loneliness and fulfills a need for both resident and pet.

Music

"Nothing brightens my wife's attitude more than our singing love songs together," stated one loving spouse who noticed how music affects his wife who has Alzheimer's disease.

"Have you ever observed persons with Alzheimer's disease, even the severely demented, and their reaction to music or singing?" asks one staff member. *"Our nursing home recently gave us, both family and staff, the pleasure of being 'entertained' by all the residents of our special care unit at Christmas time. Yes, they entertained us! Dressed in their fineries, with make up on and hair combed, they sang all the old favorites. Amazingly, even though some could no longer speak or recall the correct word name, they seemed to remember every word to the old carols and songs. One elderly gentleman even*

sang his college fraternity fight song, though he did not recognize his own wife, and mostly sat silently, humped over in his wheelchair the rest of the time."

Another family member shares:

"My elderly Dad thought another resident was his now-deceased wife. And she, in fact, thought he was her husband. They would hold hands, look into each other's eyes, and sing love songs to each other. 'Let Me Call You Sweetheart' was the song they loved the most. It generated such caring feelings between them."

Recent studies are finding scientists can now actually measure the therapeutic benefits of music. It is not clearly understood, but in studies where music was played four or five times a week, astonishing levels of change occurred:

"Most of the patients at our VA hospital where we conducted our study did not know their own names, nor recognize their spouse or children. Yet they seemed to react to music. We could see the changes and see how the men with Alzheimer's disease recognized each other, and each other's favorite music. Then the real physical proof came with the blood test. In fact, six weeks after the music-sessions study ended, melatonin levels were still more than 400 percent higher than before the music was introduced. There could be no bias in our study. Your body fluids don't tell lies," claimed a University of Miami music therapist.

It appears that as the brain deteriorates in Alzheimer's disease, the simple music of a <u>single</u> voice or a <u>single</u> instrument is the best. Many persons with Alzheimer's disease seem to like lullabies, and still others seemed to be soothed by the low beat of a single drum.

"I've even observed a foot of a severely demented person tapping to the beat of the old Glenn Miller sounds," says one therapist. Even though there is no clear understanding of how the brain processes music, there is evidence of cognition of musical sounds which elicit pleasant memories and a means of communication when all else fails.

☒

It is not unusual to find patients with Alzheimer's disease who keep singing the same song over and over. One caregiver reported, *"A resident in my unit sings 'Don't Fence Me In' over and over again. We need to see the humor in such situations because this particular little lady is a happy-go-lucky woman, who likes to converse with everyone, so her song was not one of woe and grief."*

Music therapy is becoming more and more recognized for its soothing effect on Alzheimer's patients, especially in the later stages of their disease. Research completed at the University of Kansas suggests:

"Music therapy for caregivers with their care receivers recovers that emotional closeness they seek by engaging them in meaningful participation together." Their view is that many devoted spouses desire intimacy, and music may be the catalyst to sharing an intimate moment together.

Music therapy protocol developed by board certified music therapists at a Veterans Affairs Medical Center in Topeka, Kansas, demonstrated success with integrating both caregivers and care receivers into groups. Ironically, it was not the singing that brought them together, but the physical activity of dancing, or holding each other and rocking to the music. It was concluded that music therapy was therapeutic for both the caregivers and their care receivers:

"It provided opportunities of interaction, while it contributed to the quality of the relationships, and subsequently to the quality of life for both caregivers and their care receivers. It gave caregivers and their loved ones an opportunity to be together as a couple again."

Many care plan goals include encouraging a resident to take part in sing-alongs. *"By singing the older songs from their youth, many residents show improvement in their memories by brining those old songs to mind. It also helps improve socialization of our residents,"* states one administrator.

In still another study, this one funded by the Alzheimer's Disease and Related Disorders Association, a physician relays this information:

❦

"A survey of music therapists found that music was frequently used to increase socialization, to maintain/increase cognitive skills, and to provide sensory stimulation in older populations. Music can significantly enhance the lives of people with Alzheimer's disease and can even elicit responses in the final stages of the disease."

Many such studies are currently being conducted throughout the United States, and their significance is in providing a pleasant and diverting way to stimulate long-term memories for the majority of persons with Alzheimer's disease.

For more information on music therapy, contact the National Association for Music Therapy.

Outings

"I pick up my mother from the nursing home and take her to dinner at least two times a week," declares a caring daughter. *"She cannot remember that we are going, or that we did go, so I no longer tell her ahead of time when to expect me. She always welcomes the idea with a smile and has never refused my offer. During dinner we share light conversation, talking about anything Mom wants to talk about. She almost seems 'normal' while we are out. Even though I know she never remembers our outings, she seems happy and content when I return her to the home."*

This is such an important lesson to remember. Individuals with Alzheimer's disease cannot remember things, especially the short-term memory events. The truth is, however, they retain the good feelings of the outing long after the actual memory disappears. Nursing home staff who take their residents on monthly outings report that when they return, behavior problems are greatly reduced because residents are feeling good about themselves. It seems the lingering feelings of goodness and worth remain long after the memories of the activities disappear.

"If you are wondering if it is worth it to expend the energy to take a loved one on an outing," remarks one caregiver/nurse, *"remember this: even if she doesn't know who you are, and will never remember the event, notice the smiles and joyous feelings that remain with her long after the event is over. These feelings of goodness can be better than any 'upper' medication on the market!"*

"As a Unit Director on an Alzheimer's unit, we often take some of the residents on brief outings," relates another nurse. *"The residents seem to thoroughly enjoy themselves and I have never witnessed increased confusion or difficulty in returning 'home' after the event. We invite community and family volunteers to accompany us to make sure we always have a one-to-one ratio of patient to staff/volunteers."*

"I pick my Dad up from his nursing home and take him grocery shopping with me each week," a caring daughter explains. *"He always loved to do the grocery shopping before Alzheimer's disease set in. He pushes the cart while I select items from the shelves. Sometimes I select two items and ask which one he prefers. He always enjoys these outings and is in a good mood when we return."*

"As direct care staff at a nursing home, I don't think we should be the ones who decide which residents might do well on outside outings and which will not. I know it depends on the functional level and preferences of each resident, but we found it was best to give everyone an equal opportunity, and even more than one opportunity, to see if an outing was therapeutic, or did it cause some stress. The large majority take great pleasure in our outings, returning tired, but happy."

Spiritual Needs

"Many people with Alzheimer's disease can respond to faith rituals and symbols," so say the experts who have studied such responses. Yet many families and spiritual directors ignore the spiritual needs of individuals with Alzheimer's because they fear the confusion in the person who is demented will result in failure to understand such rituals. An experienced spiritual director refutes that theory:

"I believe all people have a spiritual side which uses emotions and feelings. In my experience in working with Alzheimer's patients, I have learned it is that spiritual, feeling side that is one of the last functions to diminish. I believe most individuals with Alzheimer's disease retain their "feeling" side, thus their need for spirituality, far longer than most of us first understood."

Many caregivers believe that cognizant thoughts remain in the brains of their loved ones even when a communicative response is limited. Therefore, no one can actually know with certainty what the spiritual needs of another human being might be. Knowing how long-term memory is retained by a person suffering from Alzheimer's disease, it can be assumed that long-term beliefs are imbedded in the mind and recognized by the individual with Alzheimer's.

"Often familiar Bible verses, hymns, prayers, and even religious articles like a rosary, may elicit a memory from the past and be embraced by a person whose disease prevents him or her from communicating in any other way," shares an observant caregiver.

Visiting

Visiting people with Alzheimer's frequently presents a special challenge to family and friends. Visitors lament, "They don't even remember who I am," or "They can't carry on a normal conversation, so what should I do on a visit?" Let the person with Alzheimer's set the pace, or conversation, and take it from there. Most persons with Alzheimer's are so delighted to have you visit, they will welcome your attention whether they are in an institution or living in their own homes.

Your whole goal in visiting a person with Alzheimer's disease should be the satisfaction of leaving that person feeling good about the visit. Focus on their abilities, not their memory limitations. If they can still communicate and speak fairly well, reminisce about the past. Begin with "I remember the time. . ." Don't underestimate what the person with dementia may remember, and never contradict the way they remember. Keep in mind that long-term memory is what lingers the longest. A person with Alzheimer's may not remember if they ate breakfast that morning, but they may recall, with vivid detail, the college football game that won the championship title.

The monotony of normal, daily routines can become depressing even for persons with Alzheimer's disease. Visits from friends and relatives often interrupt this routine and provide much enjoyment.

"It is a very lonely life for the patient in a nursing home who has Alzheimer's disease. So please visit and speak to the residents," a nurses aide implores. *"A patient may not answer, but she needs to know you saw her and recognized that she did not become invisible, and is worthy of your attention."*

What to do when visiting a person who has Alzheimer's disease remains a questions on the minds of many family members and friends. Whether it be at their own home, or in a special care facility, visitors are frequently uncomfortable about what to do or what to say to a person who has Alzheimer's disease. Here are some helpful suggestions from caregivers:

"Bring in a baby to cuddle or a child to visit. Intergenerational visits can be very beneficial to both the young and old."

"Reading to a person with Alzheimer's disease is an activity that seems to be enjoyed. I would avoid complicated novels or books and stick to simple stories, or even short poems. Often the soothing voice of a child reading can be very comforting to a person with Alzheimer's disease."

"We have one family member who brings her young daughter in to visit her grandmother," says a facility administrator. *"It seems like the soothing voice of that young child reading is very comforting to her grandmother."*

Since most persons with Alzheimer's retain their need to be needed, or useful, simple chores, especially those involving repetitive actions, can be fun and stimulating during visits. These activities often promote conversation as well. Simple chores like folding socks, making a bed, watering a plant, or setting the table can provide well-needed activities for those with dementia. Research has shown the need to be needed remains long after other thoughts and feelings have diminished.

"We have a visitors' room set up for the dementia residents and their families or friends who have difficulty with communication" explains a social worker. *"This is known as our 'Senses Room' because we try to communicate peace and tranquillity through the senses. We use aroma therapy such as the recommend lavender, rosewood, or ylang ylang as calming, relaxing fragrances. As you enter the small room, you are greeted with the aroma that constitutes peacefulness and relaxation. Gentle music is playing in the background. A large lighted fish tank is set up in a darkened area that has two rocking chairs. As our residents and guests sit and rock, listening to the gentle music, smelling the relaxing aromas, and watching the fish in the lit aquarium, the feeling of tranquillity seems to quiet each of the senses and, in turn, communicates peacefulness to the soul, without words spoken."*

During a visit some family members get impatient with their loved ones and feel their visits are useless. Often the loved one with Alzheimer's disease does not even recognize the family member. It may be difficult to think of things to do or say during the visit. *"Don't stop visiting,"* implores a Patient Relations supervisor. *"It helps staff to know family members are still involved in that person's life and that your visiting is still important enough for you to take your time to do. Just being there can result in your being the advocate for your family member with Alzheimer's."*

"If visiting is feeling like wasted time, try shortening your visit and making it more structured," suggests another staff member. *"If your loved one is ambulatory, take him for a walk, outside, if weather permits. Or do some quiet activities that may elicit good feelings for your loved one. Remember, they will often not recognize who you are, or remember that you were there, but the loving feeling you show will long linger and contribute to their feeling of worth, even if they cannot express those feeling."*

"Sometimes my Mom gets agitated with the constant movement of my toddler daughter," remarks this daughter. *"It just depends on Mom's mood that day. Sometimes our visits are cut short, but I always feel like Mom is better off for our having visited, even if she doesn't remember we were there."*

"At the nursing home where my aunt is, they allow us to bring pets in to visit," explains a family member. *"It is an amazing 'therapy' she gets, and I love watching her stroke the fur of my cat. She thinks it is HER cat, and loves to talk to it like a child."*

A social worker gives the following advice on effective, creative visiting: *"Try to make certain that your expectations of the visits are realistic. Also, don't hesitate to ask the staff who cares for your loved one what type of activities might be appropriate for that individual at this stage in their disease process. Remember, it is by sharing ideas that we learn new and innovative ways to care for your loved ones who have Alzheimer's disease. On that same note, don't hesitate to offer your suggestions for activities staff can do to entertain the residents there. Together we learn!"*

Creative caregiving goes hand-in-hand with compassionate communication. Read on for further ways to enhance the caregiving experiences.

13
COMPASSIONATE COMMUNICATION

Communicating with a person who has Alzheimer's disease is one of the most discussed, yet least understood aspects of the disease. In order to establish communication, a caregiver must be willing to change his own way of thinking. The caregiver must realize a person with Alzheimer's no longer thinks the same way as a normal person. Thus a caregiver must revise verbal and non-verbal communication to a level of understanding for the person with dementia.

"We have to understand a person with Alzheimer's disease has a physical illness, not a 'mental condition' they can overcome if they just work at it," voices an understanding caregiver/spouse.

"Try not to correct everything they say, hoping the person will eventually 'get it' and be cured," cautions another astute professional caregiver.

"The most important thing in trying to communicate with a patient with Alzheimer's is to provide as normal an environment and existence as possible, with as few obstacles to memory as possible, for as long as possible," is the way this caregiver sums up compassionate communication.

In the recent past, professionals erroneously believed a concept called "reality orientation" would help the person with dementia retain their memory skills. Caregivers would continually challenge the thinking of the person with Alzheimer's by contradicting the memory loss and insisting on reality. Grueling verbal encounters resulted when caregivers were determined to help the individuals "overcome" their memory loss. This type of therapy worked for persons recovering from strokes, and it helped retrain the brain into using new thought patterns. Unfortunately, the brain cells that guide memory paths are destroyed with Alzheimer's disease and new paths are impossible. Reality orientation was theorized to be a weapon against memory loss effects. If it worked for stroke patients, it surely would work for Alzheimer's patients. In essence, reality orientation only threatened an already confused person and proved to destroy any remaining feelings of self-worth the patient might have had.

One caregiver relates this episode of "reality orientation" he observed: a social worker trying to <u>teach</u> a new resident on an Alzheimer's Unit what room she was in:

"Helen, I want you to remember you are in Room 642. Now what room are you in?" said the social worker.

"Two?" replied Helen with a questioning look on her face.

"No, Helen, you are in Room 642. Now say 'I am in room 642,'" the social worker continued.

"642," replied the compliant patient.

"That's good! Now tell me again, Helen. What room are you in?"

"Room?" asked the confused patient.

"Yes, Helen, what is your room number?"

"Number," Helen uttered while she waited for approval of her answer.

"Helen, look at me," the social worker insisted, as her voice grew more demanding. "Now say this to me: 'I am in Room 642.'"

"I am in Room 642," Helen replied as tears began to fill her eyes.

"That's perfect, Helen!" a jubilant caregiver said, believing she had *taught* Helen to remember her room number. "Tell me again. What room are you in?"

"In," whispered Helen as she looked outside the door for someone to help her.

"No, Helen, tell me your room number!" the frustrated social worker demanded once more.

"Room number," replied a very confused, frightened patient.

And so it goes—on and on. Trying to *teach* a person with

Alzheimer's disease to *remember* something is never going to work. It is imperative to understand this concept: the part of the brain that delivers short-term memory messages is destroyed in a person who has Alzheimer's disease. Forcing memory recall and laboring to get a person to retain memory, only brings frustration for the caregiver and feelings of worthlessness for the patient.

If that social worker understood a person with Alzheimer's disease does not have the capability to *remember*, the scene could have been something like this:

"Hi, Helen, my name is Martha, and I am a social worker," she could say in a lowered tone of voice, as she looked directly into the patient's eyes. "You look so pretty today," she could add with a smile and a soft touch on the patient's arm. "Come with me, Helen, to your new room?" she could direct as she held out her arm to assist the patient up. "This is your new room, Helen. It is Room 642. We will always help you find your room."

Such an encounter puts the patient at ease, orients her to person and place, reassures her of future help, accepts her memory loss as normal for her and offers the respect that person deserves.

Proper Approach

Effective communication with a person who has Alzheimer's disease begins with the initial approach. The lowered tone of voice, looking directly at the person to whom you are speaking, speaking in short phrases, and constantly reassuring the person with Alzheimer's are the proper approaches that will lead to effective, compassionate communication.

"If we just remember that mostly during the middle stages of the disease, the 'precious present' is all the memory *that remains. We need to approach the person with Alzheimer's like it is a new experience each time,"* a nurse/caregiver advises. *"Assume they will not remember having done this before or been here before. Take their lead and 'play their game'!"*

"Approach each person, each time, with dignity and positiveness," encourages this experienced nurse. *"Even though I see the same residents on my unit almost every day, I approach each one as if it is the first time we are meeting. I speak slowly, looking directly into their eyes, and always with a calm smile on my face. It is this matter-of-fact approach that puts them at ease and gives me the cooperation I need from them."*

One wise granddaughter shared this advice with caregivers:

"Patients need to know exactly what to expect and who to expect it from at the time certain care is given. By this I mean when it is bathtime, tell the patient 'I am Becky, your nurse. I have come to give you your bath.' They can remember this for the moment. But if you tell them, 'After I eat lunch, I will be back to give you your bath,' they will never remember this. So when you return to bathe them, they may resist your attempts and become afraid, because they don't know who you are or why you are taking off their clothes!"

It is important to daily, or constantly, win the trust of a person with dementia through your approach by chatting first to create a pleasant mood. Cognitive dysfunction does not mean a lack of feeling. This approach, more often than not, will make a difference in eliciting the cooperation and understanding from persons who have Alzheimer's disease.

Understanding

Most of what has been learned about communicating with those who have Alzheimer's has come from experienced caregivers, both family and professional. Doctors and nurses, administrators and social workers rarely have a specific course in their training on the care of Alzheimer's patients. There is no textbook to rely on to help caregivers understand the skill differences needed to communicate with individuals with Alzheimer's disease. Yet, according to the Alzheimer's Association, 50 percent of patients who are over the age of 85 will have dementia and will require special communication skills from the caregiver. This is precisely one of the prime reasons for writing this book: to share the information experienced caregivers have gained, in an effort to attain the understanding needed for compassionate communication.

Professionals can learn from family caregivers:

"I encourage all caregivers to LISTEN to family members regarding the care of that patient," a nurse implores. *"Most family caregivers have learned, through trial and error, just what works best in communicating with this person. Most have cared for this family member for years and are willing to share ideas and 'tips' that have worked for them. If you take the time to LISTEN to the advice of family caregivers, it can make your job easier and your patients' lives much more content."*

Another point in understanding is to become keenly aware of the words a person with Alzheimer's disease might be hearing. Never talk in front of them as if they weren't there. They may hear things that will upset them, yet they will be unable to communicate back exactly what was heard. Only the FEELING they experienced about what was heard remains (refer to Chapter 11).

One caregiver tells this story about his dear wife who has Alzheimer's disease and who had a sister named Marion:

"On a recent TV program my wife was watching, one doctor said to another, 'Marion is dead!' My sweet wife heard only those words, 'Marion is dead,' and she burst into tears, lamenting 'Marion is dead! Marion is dead!' as she put her hands to her face and cried. I tried to comfort her as I reassured her that everything was OK, and that Marion was fine. Then I distracted her to talk about Marion and the good times they shared." Caregivers, become aware of what words might elicit a lucid thought or memory for a person with Alzheimer's disease. One never knows what cognitive memory might be triggered by

the words that are suddenly heard, but not fully understood.

Compassionate communication requires caregivers to put themselves into the mindset of a person with Alzheimer's disease in order to more clearly understand how a that person "thinks." With memory brain cells depleted, thought processes take another route through the brain resulting in constant confusion. One health care administrator described it this way:

"I believe Alzheimer's disease must be like going to a new job on the first day. I'm sure you can all recall the many questions entering your mind as you approached that first day on a new job. Where is the bathroom? Where do I put my purse? When do I go to lunch? Where do I eat lunch? Who are all these people? Just imagine now, how it must be for a person with dementia. EVERY day is like this. A person with Alzheimer's disease cannot remember what was just told to him/her, or what just occurred. Each person he/she encounters is a new person with no recall of ever having met before. Each situation is a new situation, with no recall of having done this in the past."

To further enhance communication efforts, especially in the early stages, make an effort to include a person with Alzheimer's in small decisions, if feasible. The suggestion of "guided choices" is one way to help this person feel valuable by meriting a choice: "Would you like to wear this dress or that one?" "Would you like to have a cookie or ice cream?" Many people with memory loss seem to respond with appreciation for your having included them in a decision. Most likely you will know when your loved one is no longer able to make those "choices" for himself or herself.

Accepting persons with Alzheimer's disease may include an understanding of their language. Often they make up words to use in place of real words. The word used to describe the made-up words used by persons with Alzheimer's is called "neologisms." As their word-finding skills decrease, those with dementia may try to fill in the gaps with a vocabulary all of their own, or they may put a real word in inappropriate places in their sentences.

One nurse noted this incident:

"Once during an interview, I asked a resident to tell me what this is called, as I pointed to my wrist watch. With perfect confidence and a smile on her face she said it was 'A party!' I told her that is just the information I needed and she seemed pleased with herself."

Sometimes the information they give seems "off the wall" or preposterous. The number one rule in keeping the lines of communication open is this: never, never correct or ridicule a person with Alzheimer's disease who may give such an answer. In their own minds they are saying the right word. As confused and demented as they may seem, individuals with Alzheimer's disease know the feelings you mirror, and they will take that on as their own feeling. So if you have to "play the game" and accept the word "party" in place of "wrist watch," consider it another step in the process of compassionate communication.

Avoiding Arguments

Never, never argue with someone who has Alzheimer's disease. Understanding they cannot remember, the tactics of argument only cause grief and hardship for the individual with Alzheimer's. Instead, communication can be achieved through practical, creative approaches to problems that may cause such confrontations.

One caregiver shares her insight:

"My mother would insist her clothes did not need laundering and we had a fight every day as I tried to reason with her about the need to put on fresh clothing. Then a support group member told me to try this: as soon a Mom went into the bathroom, 'steal' her dirty clothing and replace them with fresh, clean clothing. It sounds so simple—but it worked! We never argue about it anymore. I had

forgotten that communication rule about never trying to reason with a person who has Alzheimer's disease."

A husband/caregiver was having difficulty convincing his wife, who has Alzheimer's disease, that they now needed to have help in the home with her daily grooming and activities. He could no longer do it by himself. He hired a nurses aide and tried to convince his wife that she needed the help of this "nurses aide." She insisted she didn't need or want help, yet it was obvious that she was unable to continue to care for her own needs. The husband then had a brain storm. His wife had been a prominent executive who had always had a "personal secretary" to assist her. He decided to <u>call</u> the nurses aide a "personal secretary" instead of a "nurses aide" and that made all the difference in attitude. The wife LOVED having her "personal secretary" come in daily; it didn't seem to matter that the "personal secretary" assisted her with her bath and grooming. The wife even introduced her aide as her "personal secretary" to her friends. Creativity can make all the difference in the responses of a loved one with Alzheimer's disease. In order to avoid arguments, go outside the realms of *your* reality and "create" the atmosphere for care that will be acceptable to your loved one.

"Keep It Simple, Sweetie" ("KISS" Principle)

The feelings of uncertainty and confusion never disappear for a person with Alzheimer's disease—they only worsen. One means of communicating is to simplify your words. Most people with early to mid-stage Alzheimer's can follow simple one-step commands if they have time to process the proper brain connections to a response. They are unable to remember more than one short statement at a time. They need a caregiver who has an immense amount of patience and is willing to give them time.

"A person with Alzheimer's disease can no longer figure out what things are for, and his normal tasks are now too complex for

X

---

his level of understanding. Simplify things for him by breaking his tasks down into very small steps," advises this caregiver.

    "Break tasks down into steps small enough for the person to handle, yet preserving the dignity an adult deserves," advises an activities director. *"Keep in mind that even if the task is something they have done numerous times per day for maybe fifty years, the complexity of a task as simple as brushing one's teeth, can be overwhelming for the person with dementia."*

Giving simple directives, without ordering, can go something like this:

"Come with me, Martha."

"We are going into the bathroom to brush your teeth."

"Here is your toothbrush, Martha."

"Put some water on your toothbrush."

"Put some toothpaste on your toothbrush."

"Brush your teeth."

"Now brush in back. Good!"

"Now brush the other side."

"Now brush the front."

"That's great."

"Spit out the toothpaste, Martha."

"Rinse off your toothbrush in the water."

"Put your toothbrush in the holder."

"Here is your cup, Martha."

"Put some water in your cup."

"Now swish your mouth with water."

"Spit out the water."

"Good!"

"Put your cup on the sink."

"Wipe off your mouth in this towel."

"Martha, come with me back to the day room."

    Most patients with Alzheimer's disease can handle such short commands and the task can be accomplished without argument or confusion on the part of the patient. It is true, however, that such care demands more time, patience, and understanding on the part of the caregiver. Yet simply saying "Go into the bathroom and brush your teeth" will result in constant reminding, arguing, and perhaps even more time. Embrace the "KISS" Principle (Keep It Simple, Sweetie) to avoid feelings of worthlessness and confusion on the part of the person with Alzheimer's who can no longer remember the "steps" of a simple task.

Validation and Distraction

The most acceptable and effective tools in communicating with a person with Alzheimer's disease are "validation and distraction." This method uses the strengths of communication a person still possesses, with the weaknesses of unavoidable memory loss. Communicating through validation and distraction basically becomes a "game," and can actually become a very pleasant and uplifting experience. This is how it is done: no matter WHAT the person with Alzheimer's says, THAT is precisely what you comment on. Validating that you HEARD what was said reassures the person with Alzheimer's of your attention and of their value as a human being. Then distracting them to a more appropriate thought/subject uses their "short memory" disadvantage to the advantage of the caregiver.

When your mother tells you she is "waiting for her husband" who died several years ago, your validation and distraction technique would be something like this:

"You really loved Pappa, didn't you?" validating you heard her comment, and then distracting her onto a pleasant thought such as, "I remember the time you went to England . . ."

"Remember that those with Alzheimer's disease have very short attention spans," this nurse/educator remarks, *"so learn to play the communication game. Take the lead from the person with Alzheimer's disease and validate and distract onto your own memories. With some practice, this routine can result in pleasant conversation and*

feelings of pleasure while dwelling on happier thoughts."

Caregivers in special care Alzheimer's units become very proficient at using the validation and distraction method:

"For the little lady-resident who comes crying to me DAILY that someone stole her purse, I assure her that we will go find that purse (validation that patient was heard) *as I lead her into the TV room and 'introduce' her to a fellow resident* (distraction)."

Caregivers can become fairly good at validation and distraction with practice. Remembering that a person with Alzheimer's disease can only concentrate on one thought at a time, you can sway that thought to one that does not cause grief or discomfort. It is up to caregivers, or even visitors, to make a person with Alzheimer's feel as comfortable and stress-free as possible. This method is a key to good communications efforts.

"Lying?"

"It seems to me the best caregivers learn to 'lie' to their loved ones who have Alzheimer's disease. I still struggle with this idea," admits a family caregiver.

Creative caregivers can get very clever at "twisting the truth" for effective communication. This often carries with it the guilt and shame of deceiving their parents or loved ones, but it is a method used to protect that loved one's integrity. It is a loving choice to change the responses for those who would only be confused by the truth.

"The best technique for minimizing the need to tell those little white lies is called 'validation.' When Mom talks about Dad who passed away ten years ago, I ask 'Are you thinking about Dad, Mom? Tell me what you're thinking about him right now.' Then when Mom replies, I will say something like, 'That makes me think about the time when you and Dad ….' What this does is validate that my Mom has feelings or thoughts about Dad, and yet not have to tell her that her thoughts are wrong because Dad died ten years ago," an experienced daughter/caregiver shares.

"I was feeling very uncomfortable about lying to my Mom who has Alzheimer's disease, so I found some good ways to avoid the truth: use distractions, use vague generalities, say 'maybe' this or that, and just simplify the truthful answer response," another caregiver resolves.

"If your discomfort level prevents you from actually lying to the Alzheimer's patient, just sort of circle around the truth," suggests this caregiver. *"We do this, not to deceive, but to bring or allow comfort to prevail. I know it makes my Mom feel much better if I don't bombard her or correct her statements with the truth. I am getting much better at playing this 'game' because I know it makes Mom feel better."*

"You should not have to resort to 'little white lies,' unless you are forced to," cautions one nurse caregiver. *"Try to use distraction with a person who has a very short attention span."*

"She kept forgetting that my grandfather passed away, and every time I reminded her that her dad was dead, she went through the pain of losing him all over again. I finally asked myself: Why am I doing this to her? She cannot remember! Why do I keep tormenting her with grief every time she asks about her dad?" questions a caregiver.

Occasionally, the "game" has to be played with any person with dementia you meet. Many caregivers have shared the experience of going into a nursing home, and one of the residents believing you are someone else—someone who has come to visit THEM. This caregiver had good advice for such a circumstance:

"An important thing to remember is that persons with Alzheimer's actually MIRROR your emotions. If you approach them with a smile and a soft voice, they will respond, often with a smile. But if you are angry or impatient with them, they will MIRROR that behavior and become angry, afraid, and most reluctant to carry on any activity you suggest. It is like a game. You meet them where they are at, whether they think you are Sally or Joan, their daughter or mother."

"If you are the spouse, the mother, or the person a loved one is calling out to, so be it," encourages a nurse/caregiver. *"BE that person he wants you to be. 'Play the game' and reap the rewards of self-fulfillment, because you alone can make this person happy if but for a brief moment. It could be all the reward you can ask for."*

"How my heart ached when I realized that my own father no longer knew who I was. After I gave myself permission to cry, and mourn the loss of the man who once recognized me as his daughter, I knew I needed to 'join his journey'," a loving daughter laments. She continues with her lesson:

"I become whomever he thinks I am, without arguing or correcting. This is so difficult, yet the single most important factor is that we are keeping the lines of communication open. If Dad thinks I am his spouse, so be it. Or if he believes I am his mother (who has been dead for 25 years!), then that is who I am. What will it hurt to acknowledge his statement and 'play the game' HIS way. It still hurts deep in my heart, but at least we can communicate, if only on HIS level."

"Many family members say they just can't 'lie' to their loved one. I say, don't lie—bend the truth for the sake of your loved one's emotions. Don't reiterate the death statement. Dwell on the LIFE of that person whom they loved so much. This can be uplifting for the whole family," one nurse emphasizes.

"Shielding a loved one with Alzheimer's disease from the truth is not 'lying,'" shares a comforting nurse. *"You don't have to be cruel with the truth either. Just do whatever is the kindest and most loving thing. Stop worrying about 'truth' or 'lies' and consider only what will make your loved one feel the best about what is being said at that moment."*

In conclusion, one empathetic caregiver summed up the debate on "lying" or twisting the truth with this explanation:

"Preserving your loved one's feelings of worth and dignity are the main reasons for twisting the truth of realty for your loved one who no longer lives in reality. Learn to play the game and do everything you can to preserve their self-worth. Feelings and emotions appear to be one of the last things to disappear in the mind. Perhaps the words get mixed up or the memory of reality is shaded, but the feelings that go along with the present moment events are what linger long after the words disappear. Do you want to leave them with a feeling of self-worth, happiness and dignity? Then don't be afraid to 'join their journey' and respond positively to all that they say. You'll reap the benefits of a happy person with a memory disorder, but one who feels good about themselves and about you."

Language Barriers

Language is another area which may compound the problems of the communication process. If a person with Alzheimer's disease knows more than one language, he will often revert back to the original language of his childhood. This goes along with the information that emphasizes how the brain retains the distant memories longer than the short-term memories. Thus the native language is retained longer than the newer language, no matter how long ago that was.

In a recent "Dear Abby" column, a spouse/caregiver wrote a letter imploring spouses of foreign-born men and women to learn the language of their spouses before communication became impossible:

"As Alzheimer's disease gradually erases the memory of the patient, starting with the present and going back chronologically to his or her childhood, the use of English or other second language disappears," wrote this husband to "Dear Abby."

He urges, *"It is important for caregivers who speak only the second language to learn enough of the patient's first language so they can communicate in basic words and phrases. I didn't; now I am faced with the complication of trying to understand the wants and needs of a French-speaking wife. Within the past six months she has regressed from all English to 75 percent French, and the change increases daily. Over the past 50 years she had lost her French almost entirely. She is as fluent today as she has ever been."*

"I deeply regret the years I rationalized that I couldn't pronounce French properly, didn't have enough time to learn it, didn't need it, and saw no future for it. So, start learning that foreign language now."

This is very valuable advice for both family and professional caregivers. Language, as a barrier, only poses more difficulties in assessment, communication, and care of those who have Alzheimer's disease.

Communicating Through Activities

Sometimes face-to-face conversations are not necessary to promote communication. The following caregivers share these creative activities as a means of compassionate communication:

"My Mom liked to look at our old photo albums, especially the really old ones from when she was a child. She would name the people and places in the pictures. I was careful not to ask her 'Do you remember. . .' That only made her agitated. So instead, it would be like telling her, and I would say 'Look, there's a picture of you and me when I was a baby!'"

"My grandmother likes to look at the greeting cards she has received, even if we look at the same ones over and over. I read them to her and then we talk about the sender, or the pictures on the cards."

"Friends save their old magazines for me to bring in when I visit my Mom. I look through them with her and talk about the pictures in them."

"I often sing to my Mom. Even though she may not recognize me as her daughter, she seems to brighten up with the words to the songs that she can remember."

"Sometimes I bring my young children to visit their grandmother in the nursing home. Since my oldest daughter is learning to read, we bring one of her simple reading books. I am amazed at how attentive my mother is when Katie reads to her. It is a fun activity for all of us

Communicating Through Touch

Another important aspect of effective and compassionate communication is that of communicating through touch. Touch is a pleasant means of communication for most persons with Alzheimer's disease and often can bring them to the reality of the task at hand. Touch seems to help "ground" a person who may be otherwise preoccupied or not cognizant of a present moment. Touch can also help calm and reassure an agitated person.

Most times a gentle touch on the arm or hand offers comfort and caring when words are not understood or communication is void. This must be approached with some discernment, however, because not all patients like to be touched. One wise nurse offers this suggestion:

"In working at the nursing home, I noticed that hugs and touch can be very warm and pleasant for most people, because most elderly people seem to be eager for hugs, gentle loving touching and hand holding. However, some do not like the invasion of their private space and prefer not to be touched. Most will tell you what they desire by their body language, and it is important to respect their boundaries."

Humor —A Means of Communication

"For me the best coping mechanism for this disease is not losing your sense of humor, and using it to communicate your love and caring," suggests this caregiver.

Humor can be the saving factor for caregivers. Recent research into humor shows that it can act as a positive force in one's life. Studies reveal that an active sense of humor can actually increase capacity for resilience, add to creativity and imagination, and even act as a barrier to stress-related dysfunction. What can be more stress-related than caring for a loved one who has Alzheimer's disease!

"*I am not telling you to laugh at a person who has dementia,*" says one caregiver. *"I am telling you to see the humor in those everyday events and share a smile and a loving hug with those who may be doing funny things."*

Laughter is actually <u>good</u> for you. It exercises your lungs, stimulates your circulation, and even exercises your breathing capacity. In addition, laughter is shown to increase oxygen in the blood, an added cardiovascular advantage.

"My mother went to button her winter coat and said, 'Oh, I am missing a button.' And then said, 'Oh, well, I'm missing my mind, too!'"

Learn to laugh with others, not at them. Adopt an attitude of playfulness, just as you adopt the "game of communication" you are learning to "play." Learn to share those humorous thoughts and observations, because laughter can actually increase relaxation.

The best kind of laughter is humor that can make light of life and all its many inconsistencies. Caring for persons with Alzheimer's disease provides many opportunities for you to look at life's contradictions, and helps you put things into perspective. Sharing these humorous moments can actually be good for you, and good for others who observe, or hear your story.

"The funniest thing that happened was when Dad put his pajama top on his legs and tried walking down the stairs. Even he shared our laughter."

"My father-in-law had been residing in a personal care facility for about six months. He had climbed over a six-foot wooden fence several times, and twice was missing for more than a couple of hours in the hot, humid Florida weather. Once, after he was returned, and after his shirt, soaked with perspiration, was changed, he said, 'Phew! I took a long walk today!'"

A granddaughter recalls with loving humor:

"She was in a store when she was still able to walk and my aunt gave her own shopping cart. All she did was go around and fill the cart with anything she could grab. It was really funny, watching her 'shopping' and all. I guess you had to be there to share a laugh."

"My Grandfather has always been a practical joker. When one of the doctors was giving the verbal tests, I had to chuckle when his reply to "Who is the President of the United States?" was an emphatic "ME!" The rest of the interview continued in the same vein. My Mother and Grandmother were both amused and aghast. We thought it was funny that Granddaddy was making fun of the banality of the questions, but knew that the doctor had not listened when he was informed of Granddaddy's penchant for tomfoolery."

"If we kept our sense of humor, the funniest thing that happened was the repetition of the same un-ending-joke that was repeated more times than could be imagined in one visit."

One professional caregiver tells this:

"I took one of our residents to the doctor and she proceeded to loudly discuss the ANATOMY of a female patient who had just come in to the doctor's office. I'll let you fill in the sorbed details of that scenario!"

Several caregivers shared these gentle scenarios in a spirit of loving humor:

"One day my mom told me that she had a long conversation with our dog."

❧

"My grandmother thought that Dick Clark from Publisher's Clearinghouse came to bring her the million dollar prize. She told everyone that everyday he came to her house and talked to her exclusively."

"I have a hard time associating funny with this disease, although I'm sure there are times that you just have to laugh and go on."

"In a dementia unit at a nursing home, a woman kept crying out, 'I want to die! I want to die!' Another patient with some humor left, shouted back, 'Somebody shoot her already!'"

"My mother gave me a pocketbook for my birthday — it was not my birthday — and she had 'shopped' for my gift in her neighbor's apartment!"

"My husband picked up my Mum from the Nursing Home for a family gathering. On arrival at the house Mum had a blue handbag (she didn't own a blue bag, and had recently been 'acquiring' other resident's belongings.) When I saw the bag I stated 'Mum, you don't have a blue bag. Where is your own handbag?' Mum said emphatically, 'Goodness, I couldn't carry a white handbag with blue shoes. Have you lost all your senses!'"

"He got irritated at me one day for one thing or another and really wanted to give me a piece of his mind. Unfortunately, the words didn't come to him and he was looking for my assistance in providing them. I suppose I could have offered up 'rotten bitch' or 'nagging witch' or something, but rather said 'You're on your own on this one, kiddo!'"

"The funniest story about things disappearing was almost four years ago when all of my Corning Ware disappeared out of the cabinet. This was just before I knew my Mom had Alzheimer's, and before I had learned how to cope. I spent weeks mentioning the Corning Ware, and the funny thing is that the lids came back. It is a joke that helps others cope with their situations. One reason is that it puts into

perspective your priorities. Someday, I'm certain I will find the Corning Ware, long after Mother is gone. If I don't, I am sure that I will survive without it."

"The most important thing to have is a good sense of humor. The things that are the most frustrating when they happen, can be a source of many laughs later. I think the ability to laugh is what saves the sanity of many caregivers."

"I asked Mom what she was doing one day as she sat in her wheelchair, oblivious to her surroundings, but mumbling and moving. She said she was 'Christmas shopping', an activity to which she had always excelled. Indeed, we found boxes of 'grandmother' gifts hidden in her closet. My sister and I were able to give these treasures to our children. It really was Christmas time, so who knows how cognizant a person really is."

"I just have to share with you the humor in listening to my <u>demented</u> *Mom and my* <u>deaf</u> *Dad conversing:*

Mom:	*"I don't know what you said."*
Dad:	*"What did you say?"*
Mom:	*"I don't know what you said."*
Dad (to me):	*"What did she say?"*
Me (to Dad):	*"She doesn't know what you said."*
Dad (to Mom):	*"I didn't say anything."*
Mom:	*"I don't know what you said "*

Humor can be fun. It's OK to laugh. Most people love to laugh. It is good for the soul. It makes everyone feel better mentally and physically. And it acts as a natural tranquilizer.

"Often if you laugh, your loved one with Alzheimer's will mirror your actions."

Smiles are "catchy." See if a smile or laughter might also elicit laughter from your loved one. You may be pleased to find that many individuals with Alzheimer's disease have the ability to retain their sense of humor long after other mental faculties have failed. So learn to laugh at life's situations.

"We caregivers don't laugh at someone, we laugh about the situation. Then we share our laughter with a friend," comments this caregiver.

Steve Allen tells us, "Nothing is better than the unintended humor of reality;" and Victor Borge once said, "Laughter is the shortest distance between two people"; or better yet, "He who laughs, lasts" —such important messages for caregivers!

Momentary Moments of Awareness

Many people with Alzheimer's disease, when their memory seems to be totally gone, live in a seemingly unreachable private world of their own. Some even mumble on and on endlessly through the day. Their voices are often hoarse from constantly verbalizing insensible thoughts. It seems to be a common, delightful event when something suddenly triggers a memory or a lucid thought for the person with severe memory loss. The surprise is that one never knows when that will occur. Suddenly, with a strong, normal voice, the person with memory loss will blurt out a completely, clearly lucid statement.

One daughter-in-law tells the story about her brilliant mother-in-law who tragically was reduced to total memory loss with her disease. She did not even recognize her own children, yet they visited her regularly and engaged her in conversation about current events. One day her son brought in a needlepoint bag that she had painstakingly worked on for over four years. She had never been the domestic type and had taken on this project long before her mother-in-law had become memory-impaired. Her husband took the bag to her nursing care room and said, "Mom, look what JoJo made for you," realizing that his Mom would surely never remember her daughter-in-law, if she didn't even know who <u>he</u> was! The mother fingered the needlework and examined it carefully and then suddenly responded, "JoJo made this for me? She doesn't even know how to sew!"

That momentary flash of full connection with the real world is an often unanticipated, yet delightful surprise for families and caregivers. Welcome it, embrace the moment, and share your delight with other caregivers, both family and professionals. It adds a bit of humor to their otherwise gloomy day and gives everyone some news to smile about as they relive that lovely moment with you.

"Even after significant progression of Alzheimer's disease, there are times when the Alzheimer's person is 'there,'" suggests one caregiver. Once more this affirms the belief of the momentary moments of cognizance. Researchers believe that many of these thoughts are "locked in" the mind of a person with Alzheimer's disease. If they are allowed to BE who they are, and families and caregivers allow them to engage in conversation, the sheer joy of sharing these times will be met with satisfaction and love.

Conclusion

Compassionate communication through your approach, validation and distraction, humor, and understanding are the only ways to make life bearable for you, the caregiver, and for the persons with Alzheimer's disease. It is sometimes called the "tricks of the trade," for it is the most sensitive, responsive approach to persons who can no longer communicate normally. Knowing and understanding the keys to communication will make the difference in your ability not only to cope, but to elicit peace and cooperation from the person with Alzheimer's disease.

14
SEEKING HELP

"In my own experience in working with families," a case manager reveals, *" it is not until they understand their own need to seek and accept the support and help of their community, that they can begin to cope with caring for a loved one with Alzheimer's disease."*

When families are learning to cope with Alzheimer's disease: groping for an understanding of the process and searching for answers, it is clear that education, counseling and support can make the difference in their courage, fortitude and survival.

The Need For Caregiver Support

A recent study reported in *The Journal of the American Medical Association (JAMA)* found that individuals who receive support and counseling while caring for a relative with Alzheimer's disease, are able to delay nursing home placement for about a year. The study revealed that caregivers in the group which received counseling and support were 82 percent less likely to put a <u>mildly</u> demented relative into a nursing home; they were 62 percent less likely to put a <u>moderately</u> demented relative into a nursing home than those in the non-supported group. This study sustains the theory that education and support of the caregiver are key to the success of caregiving.

Most all communities today offer Alzheimer's educational programs, support, and counseling for families and caregivers coping with Alzheimer's disease. There is a national Alzheimer's Association for referrals and support. There are various local agencies that offer information and support. The most important emphasis for caregivers from such agencies is to know and understand their own need for help.

Whether it be formal, professional help, support group sharing, or the assistance of a caring neighbor, the message of the need for caregiver support is always evident. Here are the "voices of experience": caregivers who offer their advice about seeking help.

Where To Begin

A wise counselor for caregiving family members shares this advice:

"You as a caregiver must understand you have to take care of yourself. Becoming exhausted or ill taking care of a loved one with Alzheimer's disease compounds the problem. I would first suggest that you find the many resources offering tips for caregivers. These will be through Alzheimer's Associations, the library, support groups, even the Internet. Learn all you can. These tips will help you cope with the situation. Then make certain that your loved one has a complete physical and psychological workup by a reputable physician. Third, check the Yellow Pages for home health agencies and adult day care centers which may be able to assist you. Most agencies have social workers or case managers who will assess your loved one and assist you with financial considerations. Then, please, please accept the help that is offered."

"When we first suspected Dad might have Alzheimer's disease, we were terror-stricken," a daughter related. *"A friend recommended we call the Alzheimer's Association. We were referred to our local chapter and they couldn't have been nicer or more informative. They started by helping us find a place for Dad to be evaluated. It turned out we were right, it WAS Alzheimer's disease. Then the organization continued with their incredibly sympathetic and supportive information about care facilities and support groups for us. It was such a positive experience for us—and a growing one. They all helped us find our way through the MAZE of health care to assess exactly what services our Dad needed."*

Listed here are some of the organizations which can help caregivers begin their search for assistance:

The Alzheimer's Association has a toll-free number:
1-800-272-3900
The Alzheimer's Association will provide the phone numbers and locations of local resources. They will send free information and resources for education. The Alzheimer's Association was founded in 1980 and is the only national voluntary health organization dedicated both to research for the causes, treatments, cures and prevention of Alzheimer's disease, as well as to provide education and support for people with the disease, their families and caregivers. The Alzheimer's Association has a network of more than 200 chapters in 50 states working with over 35,000 volunteers providing programs and services to assist those with the disease and their families. A nationwide 24-hour information and referral line links families who need assistance with nearby Chapters.

The Alzheimer's Disease and Referral Center at 1-800-438-4380 is an additional resource for information and education about Alzheimer's disease.

Every state also has an Area Agency on Aging which has networks of provider services for the elderly at the city, county, and/or multi-county levels. Staff are prepared to help caregivers with any problems and make referrals to local resources. See your local phone directory for the number in your state.

Another informative resource is:
The National Council on Aging
1-800-375-1014
This organization is an association of some 7000 groups and

individuals committed to promoting the dignity, self-determination, well-being, and contribution of older persons. It serves as a national resource for service providers and consumers. Special areas of interest are community-based programs, including senior centers and adult day services. Several helpful pamphlets are available on adult day care and independent living facilities offering assistance ideas for elders to stay in their own homes longer.

For those who have Internet access to the World Wide Web, the following websites will be helpful:

The Alzheimer's Association   www.alz.org
Caregiver Network   www.caregiver.on.ca/
The Alzheimer's Page   www.biostat.wust1.edu/alzheimer/

Please note that not all Alzheimer's associations are members of the national organization, so check with your local hospitals, senior services, or phone listings for the resource center nearest you. Most organizations offer free services and information to caregivers. Besides support group information, many have a monthly newsletter, a resource center, and information hotlines for handling difficult behavior. Many of them are staffed by people who are, or have been, caregivers themselves.

Support Groups

No information about Alzheimer's disease and caregiving is complete without referrals to a support group. Some may have an erroneous view of what an Alzheimer's support group is or be leery of attending. Here, in their own words, experienced caregivers offer these insights:

"Support groups are for the caregivers. Support groups are the number one place for caregivers to cry, to learn, to share, to help,

and even to laugh together. Caregivers help one another to take an honest and realistic look at the situation, and to provide the best help and advice possible: the words of experience. This is the place where <u>caring for the caregiver</u> takes precedence."

"Caregivers for those with Alzheimer's need to come together at least monthly to network and share with those who understand best their problems and frustrations. Many support group facilitators are or were caregivers themselves. Some facilitators are professionals. All that is needed for a support group is a place to meet and a person who would be willing to coordinate the meetings."

"There was, and is, a great need for support groups," one facilitator attests. *"They can be a lifesaver to someone who is dealing with the behavior of Alzheimer's patients. We have had more than 30 people attend our group. The caregivers who attend are caring for patients from very early stage (not diagnosed) to the final stages. They range in age from 30 to 95. The input from these people is invaluable in learning new skills to handle problems as they arise."*

No formal agenda is necessary for a support group unless the group desires that. Support groups give each caregiver time away from their loved one with Alzheimer's, and time to learn new ideas for care. It should be a safe place for caregivers to cry and even to laugh. It is a "meeting of the hearts" and can be most uplifting. This is what caregivers have to say about their experiences in a support group:

"My Mom, who cares for Dad who has Alzheimer's disease, finally attended a support group meeting. She found it to be just what she needed: people like her. She found someone to lean on, someone to call on when she needs to talk. I am so glad she found them."

"Holding hands is a good way to go through life, and that's what we do through our support groups. It helps us get through the difficult periods and lets us know we are not alone."

"As a nurse professional, the best advise I can give caregivers is to stick with a support group. Sometimes you will be helped. Sometimes your experience will aid others. But most of all, support groups help you take care of yourself. If you don't, who will?"

"There is no doubt support groups allow caregivers to form bonds among themselves as they meet together on a regular basis. They have an opportunity to share with others who understand, first hand, their feelings, concerns, and problems. Many actually become close friends and carry on that friendship long after the mutual circumstances that first brought them together have changed."

A young wife whose husband had been diagnosed 14 years ago, at the age of 50, shares this insight:

"I hesitated joining a support group because I thought it would mean sitting around with a bunch of crybabies. How wrong I was! The members were caregivers too. They knew first-hand exactly what was going through my mind. We help each other. They're like family to me now. I can phone one of them at any hour if my husband's illness becomes too much for me to bear."

"Caregivers, you have a RIGHT and an obligation to take time for your own support without feeling guilty. If it comes down to whether a decision about attending a support group is better for you or for your loved one, choose the one that will keep you the most sane, patient and loving. You need to develop a new life for yourself, different from the one you shared with your loved one. You are the only one who can do that, and caregivers at a support group meeting can help you to do that. The art of caregiving lies in the fact that one has learned the proper balance between giving care and taking care of oneself. Ask your fellow caregivers to help you find this balance."

The following caregivers share what they have learned through their support group meetings:

"'How long will this caregiving last?' I used to ask at my support

group meeting. A kind person I met there told me it is best to prepare oneself for the long haul; try to remain flexible for the situation can be continually changing. She also said to try to always have the needs of the Alzheimer's patient be part of your life, but never all of your life.. She was right."

"My message is: YOU CANNOT DO IT ALONE. I tried for seven years, because back then there was little help available. I could not afford the high cost of home care. My income dwindled to below poverty level because of my caregiving duties. I didn't know about the Alzheimer's Associations. Today, the Alzheimer's Associations have done a wonderful job of educating the public and helping to improve and extend their services throughout the United States. I have learned about day care centers who now routinely admit Alzheimer's disease sufferers, and things are much, much better for me. The only problems I see for other caregivers are being in denial and negativity in seeking out help. Today there is no excuse not to find the help you need."

"I started to go to a local support group some time before I made the decision to move my mom into a small, residential board and care home. It was tremendously helpful to have the support of the group as I was making decisions. As for guilt, I have little. I have done, and am doing, the best I can with a lousy situation—and my support group helps me to see that each time we meet."

A nurse and family caregiver, who went through ten years of working while simultaneously caring for her mother, ended up with numerous health problems as a result of not caring for herself during that time. She is still trying to deal with the guilt of past decisions through counseling. She encourages all to learn from her mistakes, to benefit from the poor self-care decisions from her past:

"Learn to prioritize. Yes, you love your parent or spouse, but you also have other responsibilities and one of them is to care for yourself. The person you are caring for will eventually die of their disease. Hopefully you will be here for a good long time afterwards.

Take care of yourself now. If you feel burned out or even just tired, get respite. Demand it from other siblings if you need to, or arrange it through a neighbor, day care, or nursing home. Use the help that is offered freely though support groups. I am still paying for refusing help when I needed it. Don't make the same mistakes I made!"

"With my Mom's diagnosis of Alzheimer's disease, our family was devastated. We needed help to understand this disease and what might happen to her. We were totally unprepared to take on the role of family caregiver. Support groups and resource centers provided us the legal, financial, and educational help we needed, as well as training for handling difficult behavior and coping with our own emotional reactions to the changes."

"An elderly wise women once told me, 'You can't whistle a symphony.' What did she mean? It means that we cannot, I don't care how good or emotionally stable we are, get through the caregiving of a person with Alzheimer's disease all by ourselves, and come out OK. We NEED one another."

One adult child caregiver boldly expresses her feelings:

"I wish others would understand that it is not fair to condemn us when we watch confusion and distrust replace the strength and independence we once knew of this parent, and we wish for a swift end to this destruction. Such thoughts are not cruel or unusual for us. At least my support group helped me validate these previously unspoken feelings."

One caregiver describes how she leaned on her group members to deal with her grief:

"We begin to grieve at the time of the diagnosis, but feel we must keep a good front for our loved one and the family. We try to not grieve, or, if we do, we try to not let it show. Each step of the disease brings more and more loss, and more and more pressure to be positive and not lose control. If we grieve in private, we begin to bury our

feelings. Gradually we become exhausted and numb. That is why support groups are so valuable. It is a place where we can let go and express our feelings without guilt, at the time we are experiencing them. Other caregivers accept our feelings and let us know that we are normal and not crazy. We need to know that it is all right to feel sorry for ourselves and our losses. We need to have the understanding of others who have made this journey before us."

"There are no real guideposts for dealing with this disease. There are general thoughts, but no one can tell me 'Your mother is this far along in the process, and this is what will happen next, and in a year she'll be like this, and here is the next step for you to take.' This is precisely why my support group is so important to me. True, no one can tell me the course of this disease, but those who have 'been-there, done-that,' can share their wisdom and experiences to help me deal with MY present situation."

"I attend a family support group in my church. I believe family support is crucial in Alzheimer's disease care to reduce stress and help families maintain a high level of patient care. This keeps families together longer, delaying costly placement in nursing homes."

"My Mom is in the early stages of Alzheimer's disease and I'm learning how to approach everything by talking with other caregivers at weekly support group meetings. Before these meetings I had very little knowledge about the progression of this disease, yet I know this was the easy part. I can't imagine how rough it's going to get. So if I can at least get things into perspective now, with the help from my group, I'll be in a better position to handle the later stages."

"In addition to my support groups, I try to maintain outside interests and activities. I plan one non-Alzheimer's activity each week. I learned this from other caregivers in my support group."

"'Go back to your exercise program!' my support group friends told me. So I try to maintain my pre-caregiving exercise routines.

Sometimes I ask a friend, neighbor or family member to stay with my husband while I go for a walk."

"People need people and caregivers need caregivers. Sometimes I am a giver and sometimes I am a taker, but my support group has given me the help I need. I could never repay them, so I just pass on the wisdom I have gained."

" I have met some wonderful people in my support group. It's great to have some people care about ME. It makes me want to help others."

"It is very important to have a support system. If you can't find a support group near you, then by all means start one," this caregiver encourages. *"Even if you start it for selfish reasons like I did (I needed it!), it will be worth the little amount of time and effort it takes."*

"In February of 1996 I started a support group for caregivers of Alzheimer's and other dementia patients. There was not one in my town, even though the population is close to 200,000. It is a gift I gave myself—and it keeps on giving, as we help one another through some very trying times."

"I am always in awe of the many volunteers, mostly spouses, who remain year after year, to help, support, encourage and teach those of who are currently struggling with the care of a loved one with Alzheimer's disease. It is to these people we owe the biggest gratitude. For it is in their willingness to share that we have learned the most about the CARE of persons with Alzheimer's disease."

What better affirmation of the need for support groups than from the words of caregivers who share their own personal experiences and testimonials.

Support Groups For Early-Stage Alzheimer's

In addition to support groups for caregivers, because of the earlier diagnosis of Alzheimer's disease, individuals with this diagnosis are seeking information and support for themselves.:

"Many people with early Alzheimer's disease cannot work any longer. Friends have disappeared. Maybe we've begun to feel like a nuisance around the house. A support group for early-stage Alzheimer's offers an opportunity for us to meet with others like ourselves. We can help each other to see there is still a lot of living to be done. Our support group can inspire us to press on," comments this early-stage Alzheimer's support group member.

"In some cities the Alzheimer's Associations are receiving funding for support groups for persons in the early stages of Alzheimer's disease," one nurse explains. *"They often provide a broad range of medical, recreational, social and financial information to assist families and patients themselves in planning and evaluating the progress of the disease process. Many meet on a weekly basis and provide the tools to help early Alzheimer's individuals cope in an atmosphere of acceptance and with an opportunity to take part in activities that provide them with not only enjoyment, but with dignity and pride. Participation is strictly voluntary, but it takes the focus off the disability and focuses on the abilities of a person for as long a possible. Fees vary, depending on the area, but in our area, the fee is $20.00 per day which includes lunch."*

"We formed an early-diagnosed Alzheimer's disease support groups for the purpose of helping the patients with sharing sadness and trying to come to terms with the disease," another care provider shares. *"In the future we hope to offer support groups for socializing, learning how to establish routines to make life easier, or discussing plans for the future."*

One member offers this insight:

"We all have fears, you know. We're worried about the day that will come when they have to put us in a box, or whatever they do with people who can't think or speak anymore."

"It was quite a relief to find that the other people in the group weren't a bunch of morons, as I sometimes considered myself to be," stated another member. *"They are lovely people, even with their illness. There is a huge sense of loss that we all have, and many fears, but then we come here and realize we are not alone. We can let down our guard."*

One Alzheimer's patient in a support group shares this view:

"Many members see our support group as a refuge: a place where we are learning to lose our minds with dignity and humor."

A wife/caregiver comments about the support group for her young husband who has Alzheimer's disease:

"His world hasn't shrunk, his role in it has. His support group helps fill the void, so much so that my husband's week has to be defined by the meeting."

"These days, a good day is when Dad is with his support group," a daughter shared. *"He then has the feeling that life's OK. Nobody's cheering, but at least it's OK."*

"How good it is to know that I am not really alone," is the way one person who has Alzheimer's disease sums it up.

Respite Care

RESPITE. This word takes on new significance and meaning to every caregiver of a person with Alzheimer's disease. Respite can be defined as "temporary rest." It refers to "time off" for a primary caregiver to get much needed rest and a break from his/her duties as caregiver. The Alzheimer's Association defines respite care as "a necessity for every caregiver."

There are basically three types of respite: short-term stays in a nursing home or care facility, adult day care, or in-home help. Every Alzheimer's support group emphasizes the need for caregivers to seek respite <u>before</u> they get ill, depressed, or out of control themselves.

"Caregiving of a person with Alzheimer's disease becomes a 36-hour-a-day job. I am referring to a book about being an Alzheimer's caregiver, called 'The 36-Hour Day.' If there is one message I can give in loud, clear words to caregivers, it is this: CAREGIVERS, <u>SEEK RESPITE</u> BEFORE YOU NEED IT," cautions a social worker.

Many caregivers give the excuse that "I could never put my loved one in a place like a nursing home!" or "She isn't that bad yet," or, the scariest one: "I'm coping all right." But are you?

"Does coping mean you have not yet reached the end of your rope?" asks a counselor. *"Does coping mean you are too proud to recognize you need help? Does coping mean you will go on this way until you have a nervous breakdown, a serious physical happening, or totally lose it with your loved one? Of course not. Coping means you will take care of your loved one the very best way possible. And that, dear caregivers, means taking very good care of yourselves. Because if you get ill, or suffer an emotional breakdown, who will care for your loved one? Often this leads to a caregiver totally unfamiliar to the patient. So do yourself and your loved one a favor by allowing him or her to become more familiar with another caregiver."*

One family wrote about their father who single-handedly cared for their mother who had Alzheimer's disease. His children saw his health declining and felt helpless. The daughter laments with grief:

"They were a proud, upper-class couple who would not let us help and struggled alone with my mother's memory problems for years. Unfortunately, the physician never saw the signs on the wall, nor suggested respite care for my father. My father died prematurely, his

health deteriorating from the fatigue and stress of caring for mother by himself. I live with the guilt and grief of knowing that respite care may have given my Dad extra years, and may have saved my mother from the distress and depression of his death which ultimately put her into a psychiatric unit. We lost the opportunity for respite care. We are left with broken hearts and hind-sighted questions."

A case worker offers this comment:

"If care of a person with Alzheimer's disease is to continue indefinitely in the home, it is essential for caregivers to get a regular break from the daily demands imposed by this disease. Everyone benefits, including the person with Alzheimer's who gets a refreshed caregiver daily."

In addition, recent research has proven respite care is actually beneficial to the person with Alzheimer's disease. Statistics are showing that being with persons other than the caregiver can be stimulating and can often help relieve depressions and build self confidence for the person with Alzheimer's disease.

"We have a respite program through our local Alzheimer's Association. Our respite caregivers are volunteers who must take a certain number of training hours and are then assigned to a certain Alzheimer's patient to give the primary caregiver respite time. The Association does not charge a fee for these volunteers. They suggest the caregiver pay their mileage, and/or donate to the association if they are able. No one is ever denied services because they cannot afford it," one volunteer relates.

"I encourage you to take the opportunity to look into your area's respite services. Call your local Alzheimer's Association, churches, or senior clubs. Many agencies offer these services at reduced or free rates. The best way to find out about respite is to attend your local support group meetings. You then also have the opportunity to discuss with other caregivers their likes or dislikes of services available.

Many local Alzheimer's associations' staff will actually accompany you to specific day care centers or nursing homes for your first-hand observations before making your decision about respite care. Please seek the help that is available in your area," urges a family counselor.

Financial/Legal Consultants

In addition to the emotional and spiritual help support groups and respite care will provide, it is important to seek the legal and financial advice of professionals. Elder Law Attorneys specialize in legal matters to protect senior citizens and their families. Certified Financial Planners (CFP) will help organize and plan financial matters of the present and future for the individual with Alzheimer's disease and his or her family. Many support groups host these professionals as informational speakers for their members. It is also prudent to ask other caregivers for their recommendations of legal and financial consultants who have been helpful to them. Several of these professionals specialize in working with the elderly and their families.

15
UNDERSTANDING CARE OPTIONS

This final chapter is a summary of the vast array of services and housing alternatives available for those who have Alzheimer's disease. There no reason for any family member, professional, student, or friend who cares for a person with Alzheimer's disease to be without resources of information to help guide their decisions about care options and placement of these loved ones. The following explanations will aid in the understanding of available care options and offer advice of caregivers regarding such choices.

Geriatric Case Managers

Geriatric Case Managers are a team of professionals who can help and direct the family in assessing the present needs and concerns for the person with Alzheimer's disease and for the family involved in his/her care. They are a good starting point in determining the type of care needed. Many work in agencies which cater to the needs of the elderly. They can be the liaison between family needs and community resources.

Studies demonstrate that today many elders have outlived their informal support systems once provided by spouses, siblings, other relatives and friends. Many senior citizens require non-medical type care such as meals, chores, laundry and companionship which can be offered in their own homes.

"It is important to consider all alternative measures of care before making a decision about the placement of a loved one with Alzheimer's disease," one caseworker explains. *"Geriatric case managers provide this service of assessment for families."*

"Often times families are not familiar with the nursing home industry and/or other residential care options available to them,"

another case manager comments. *"They may believe there are only two choices: their own home or an 'old folk's home' which many elders believe is the place they go to die. Today we need to assist our families with education about the many alternatives to nursing homes. From homemaking/chore services in the home to assisted living, to hospice services, there is a service or facility that is right for them. My job as a Geriatric Case Manager is to find that placement or service that best meets their needs and financial situations. With the proper services, many elderly folks with Alzheimer's disease are able to remain in their homes, even when total care becomes necessary."*

Caring For Your Loved One at Home

The one place where families most prefer to care for their loved one with Alzheimer's is at home. Whether it means moving into their loved one's home, or moving the loved one in with them, most families seek this care option for as long as feasible. They believe their loved one with Alzheimer's disease will function best in an environment that is loving and supportive, and one that allows for individualized care for as long as possible. In most cases, that choice of care is home.

As demonstrated in the previous chapters, caring for someone who has Alzheimer's disease is one of the most stressful and demanding jobs encountered. Most often it is the eldest daughter or spouse of the eldest son who assumes this responsibility. Often it is an elderly spouse who finds the burdens of caregiving so demanding, it leaves him or her exhausted and a target for ill health. Frequently it is an adult child, still raising her own family at home, who becomes a caregiver.

Fortunately, there are many in-home care programs which provide respite, support, education, and/or training for at-home caregivers. Various support groups as mentioned in the previous chapter are essential in helping caregivers make the necessary adjustments, physically and emotionally, to care for a loved one at home. In addition, support groups and Alzheimer's Associations can be instrumental in guiding the caregivers to additional help and services as the situations are warranted.

If caring for a loved one with Alzheimer's disease in your own home is your family's choice, be certain to refer to the previous chapter on the necessity of caregiver support groups and respite care.

Home Health Care Services

Home health care, which offers help with needs like bathing, cooking, and/or medical/nursing treatment, is the fastest-growing segment of the health-services industry today, with some 20,000 agencies. Medicare does not cover the cost for Alzheimer's care, as it is still considered "custodial" and not "medical" services as defined by Medicare coverage restrictions. Private pay is often the only means to attain such services for a person with Alzheimer's disease. If no medical/nursing care is required, assistance with other tasks may be attained through homemaking services.

Homemaking Services

In-home homemaking services provide solutions for individuals or couples who prefer to remain in their own homes. It is designed as a non-medical, non-nursing service for people who are capable of managing their own physical needs, but who require limited assistance with light housekeeping, respite, meals or companionship. They do such things as plan, cook, and serve meals; light housekeeping duties, laundry, and errands; assistance in grooming, dressing and light exercising; and also act as a liaison between the family members and the couple or person with early Alzheimer's disease. Most are available under private pay arrangements, for from a few hours to as many as 24 hours per day, seven days a week.

"I believe if there were some type of subsidy or tax consideration for non-medical home care, we could keep our loved ones from going into nursing homes long before they really need skilled

nursing care," supports a home-care advocate.

"Most of all, caregivers and families must realize when they cannot give adequate care by themselves any longer and look toward a service or facility that can provide that care," urges a realistic caregiver.

Day Care/ Day Stay Programs

An adult day care center can be the answer for families who are seeking a safe, nurturing environment for their family members with Alzheimer's disease. Most also provide an opportunity for enjoyable, stimulating activities on a daily basis. A good day care center offers the person with Alzheimer's disease an opportunity to "belong" and to feel self worth. Chapter 12 on Creative Caregiving demonstrated how many persons with Alzheimer's disease believe they are going to a "club" or to "volunteer" or help "those older people," instead of their families calling it "going to day care."

For many years, the term "day care" referred to those centers where parents who worked left their children to be cared for by other adults. Child day care centers at first were viewed as a poor substitute for supervision of children. Studies now indicate that day care provides social and educational benefits to children whose parents need to work. We need to look at the benefits of adult day care centers the same way. They should not be the "last resort" for families who are overwhelmed with care.

A day program Recreation Therapist shared this:

"I wish the community realized persons afflicted with Alzheimer's disease can still understand what is happening around them. It is important that families be supported by the community and allow for victims to live at home and be independent for as long as possible. Nursing homes are not always the best alternative. Day programs offer respite for the caregiver and recreation for the participant. We are not a baby-sitting service and we encourage

participants to express themselves and socialize in a safe and structured environment. Alzheimer's disease is a devastating disease for both the victim and the family. It is important that both receive the support that they need."

"Day care offers increased social stimulation and activities geared to the correct level of functioning," another counselor advocates. *"This will often help to calm the person who struggles with the embarrassment of memory loss, not to mention the much needed respite for the caregiver."*

"Costs of day stay programs vary, but many offer the first day free, or at a reduced rate. It costs much less than a nursing home, and you are free to choose the number of days you want to participate. They are run by a caring staff who are not only trained, but they enjoy doing what they do," adds one director.

"Remember that the biggest problem of those with Alzheimer's disease is memory, so each new day at the center will seem like the first day. Be patient and understanding and repeat the same reason for going each day."

"It is like meeting a new friend each day, because each day at the day care center will be like the first. However, if the warm feelings of love, caring and contributing replace the ugly feelings of being a burden, being frightened or frustrated, then day care will be the place that they WANT to be, and not HAVE to be," suggests one day care center administrator.

Decisions about Care Facilities

The decision to move a loved into a care facility is one of the most difficult decisions facing families. Not only the decision to make the change, but the understanding of the many choices from the array of options can be confusing. The following list will provide information about the various levels of care:

Independent Living Facilities or Retirement Communities

Most retirement communities have medical criteria which prospective residents must meet in order to be accepted into the community. An Independent Living Facility refers to a larger complex with self-contained units, apartments or condominiums for older adults who are able to care for themselves. These facilities offer numerous amenities including organized social programs, meal service plans, housekeeping, maintenance, transportation services and emergency call bells for assistance if needed. The community may also provide varying levels of medical care based on the need for additional assistance. Couples who have one spouse with Alzheimer's disease may live comfortably for years in such an independent care facility if the well-spouse can care for the spouse with Alzheimer's disease, or if they hire in care assistance as needed.

Continuing Care Retirement Communities

Continuing Care Retirement Communities offer multi-levels of care from independent living, to assisted, to nursing home care plus an extraordinary range of services. Most have convenient buy-in or rental payment plans. Many of the buy-ins offer up to 90% refunds in the event of death or transfer. Some are called Life Care Communities because once you qualify for admission, all levels of care are included in your contract with some minor adjustment of fees. Life Care Communities offer the services, but often with complex financial implications. It is important to thoroughly understand the financial obligations of a Life Care Community. Whatever the choice, be sure to shop before the need is acute, because most times there is a waiting list. Check the Yellow Pages listings under Retirement Communities or use the Internet Index of America's Guide to Retirement Living and Senior Care (www.americasguide.com) for all such listings in the United States, by category, state, region, and city.

It will take some time to find the facility that best meets not only the present needs, but the future needs of your loved one with Alzheimer's disease. Moving from one facility to another may cause added confusion and regression for a person with Alzheimer's disease. Also think geographically. Is it important to have this loved one is a warmer climate? in a area closer to one family member than another?

Assisted Living Facilities

Assisted Living Facilities (ALF), formerly known as Adult Congregate Living Facilities (ACLF), refers to a senior community that offers both types of care environments: custodial care such as housekeeping and meals, as well as daily living assistance with bathing, medications and monitoring of activities. These types of facilities are for those who are neither fully dependent, nor fully independent on others for their care. Assisted living provides limited personal care assistance and 24-hour-a-day supervision, in an apartment-like setting. The goal here is to maximize privacy and independence, while matching the person's needs and life style against the house rules and supervision. For persons in the middle to later stages of Alzheimer's disease, this may not provide the maximum supervision needed, especially for those who wander. There are special care assisted living facilities specifically for those with Alzheimer's disease.

Average daily costs for assisted living runs about $72, and most costs are not covered by Medicare. It is important to be sure to understand exactly what services are covered for the monthly fees. Some states allow minimal public assistance in the form of Medicaid, to cover some expenses of assisted living for the elderly. Each assisted living facility should have a license to operate from a regulatory state agency defining the level of care provided.

An independent agency sponsored by the American Association of Homes and Services for the Aging (AAHSA), evaluates the top continuing care and retirement communities in the nation. You can reach them at:

Continuing Care Accreditation, 901 East Street, NW; Suite 500; Washington, D.C. 20004-2037; (202)783-7286. The Assisted Living Federation of America (ALFA) represents over 4000 facilities and offers consumers guides on choosing an assisted living facility in any area. They can be reached at 10300 Eaton Place, Suite 400, Fairfax, VA 22030.

Residential Care Facilities

Residential Care Facilities often refer to smaller assisted living facilities with a licensed capacity of six to twenty older adults. These may also be referred to as "Board and Care Facilities," "Sheltered Living," "Catered Living," or "Rest Homes," depending on the area of the country in which you live.

Nursing Homes and Rehabilitation Centers

Finding the right nursing home requires comprehensive investigation and careful viewing of each facility. Is it clean? Are the residents cared for, wearing clean clothing, and conversing with one another and with staff? Is the air free of odors? Is the staff aware of your visit and do they acknowledge you? What is the staff ratio and how does that compare with other facilities in your area? A bare minimum staff ration would be one staff member per seven patients during the daytime, and never less that one to twelve patients at night.

Nursing homes are for patients with many varying needs. Unlike the nursing homes of yesteryear, many skilled nursing facilities today offer short term rehabilitation following hospitalizations. Yearly charges can run as high as $60,000.

The Social Security Act which mandates the licensing and federal standards of care for this category refers to Nursing Homes now as Skilled Nursing Facilities (SNF). These facilities provide nursing services for those with long-term illnesses. Many also provide rehabilitation services for short-term care following a hospital discharge or for respite care. Costs vary around the country, but average $2000 to $3000 per month. Most often Medicare does not cover care for long-terms, but Medicaid or private long-term care insurance can apply.

One key to providing a continuity of care after placement is to make certain that, as family members, you know who the key people are in the facility. Some nursing homes have a staff member who serves as the liaison. Often this person is a social worker. In addition, at least monthly care meetings should be attended by a family member, the nurse in the facility, social worker, physical therapist or occupational therapist, as needed, and any other person involved in the care of your loved one. It is this meeting that the "team" of caregivers identifies problems, needs, and begins implementations of plans for the coming month. Of course, if an urgent need arises any time before the planned meeting, do not hesitate to make your needs known to prominent staff. You, family members, are the voice for the loved one with Alzheimer's disease who can not speak in their own behalf.

Patient Rights

"I needed information on patient/family rights for people who have been placed in nursing homes. This is what I discovered and wanted to share with your readers: The National Citizens Coalition for Nursing Home Reform has led the way for the past decade in advocating for nursing home residents' rights. They even have a Website at http://aginet.com/nccnhr/ *In addition, all states have ombudsman programs that work with residents to protect their rights. Check your state office for the telephone numbers."*

"When it comes to Alzheimer's patients' rights, we all have reason to justify. We all have an obligation to be advocates, too. We all must be advocates for those who may no longer be able to advocate for themselves. It is our duty as staff and family members. We need to work together."

Secured Facilities

Some facilities promote themselves as "secured" or "locked" facilities. They usually have units with locked doors at each exit, preventing residents from getting out. The security of a loved one in a facility is more a result of good staff observance and care, than it is a lock on the doors. Sometimes in large facilities with inadequate staff, patients are seen banging on the locked doors, after crying to get out. It is a wise and caring staff who is able to spend time with the resident who is insisting on leaving. Often a staff that is trained in offering some loving reassurance followed by a distracting direction will alleviate the problems at the locked door. Another hint was suggested in the "camouflaging" the doors through color. If the walls and doors are all the same color, they do not tend to "stand out" and beg a person with Alzheimer's disease to try to "escape." It is advisable to check out the safety and assurance of "secured units."

"The Eden Alternative" — A New Paradigm of Care

"The Eden Alternative" is a book and philosophy of care developed by Dr. William Thomas which identifies a concept of creating a "human habitat" in place of the nursing home. His philosophy espouses nursing home residents are not only cared for, but give care. With the initiation of pets, children and plants, residents combat loneliness, avoid boredom, have a purpose in living, and feel they are contributing members of society. Animals such as dogs, cats, and birds roam the premises and provide the stimuli that enhances life itself. Development and nurturing of plants and flowers provide the impetus needed to calm some residents by offering an environment which encourages replacing sedating drugs with calming holistic activities.

The mission statement of the Eden Alternative states that they believe they have "a powerful tool for improving the quality of life for people who live in long term care facilities. . . We teach ourselves to see nursing homes as habitats for human beings rather than institutions for the frail and elderly. . . We want to show others how companion animals, the opportunity to care for other living things, and the variety and spontaneity that mark an enlivened environment can succeed where pills and therapies fail."

Through his research at Chase Memorial Nursing Home in New York, Dr. Thomas found his method significantly reduced the need for mind-altering and mood-altering drugs. In addition, in the first year the nursing home also reduced its mortality rate by 15 percent, and the second year the rate dropped by 25 percent. In that one facility, this meant eight people were alive who otherwise would have died. It also reduced staff turnover by 26 percent because people felt better about working there.

Dr. Thomas believes, "The differences in death rates can be traced to the fundamental human need for a reason to live. No one ever told me in a medical school that doing something about loneliness, helplessness and boredom, could have a bigger impact on mortality than I can have with my prescription." Efforts are now under way to "Edenize" nursing homes in Missouri, Texas, and other states.

Alzheimer's Special Care Facilities

Because of the intense need, with over 4 four million Americans with Alzheimer's disease, many facilities are dedicating whole units, or building separate buildings, to care for persons in various stages of Alzheimer's disease. These are specialty units which offer a safe and secured environment, with specially trained staff specifically to care for persons with dementia.

In 1992, the Alzheimer's Association published a guide for establishing Special Care Units (SPU). They emphasized the need for these five features to make them qualified SPU for the Alzheimer's resident: selected residents with mild to moderate progressive dementia, specialized staff trained in the care of the Alzheimer's resident, special activity programs and environments for the cognitively impaired, and family programming and involvement.

Over the past decade the concept of special care units to meet the difficult and challenging needs of persons with Alzheimer's disease has emerged. Many debates and research studies have been undertaken to asses the value of these special care units over the traditional integrated nursing home facilities. Many health care providers support the concept of creating an environment that provides specialized care for persons with Alzheimer's disease. This is mostly because many of the traditional nursing home units were inadequate to meet the safety, environmental and cognitive needs of the residents who exhibited symptoms of Alzheimer's disease. In addition, the traditional units often were noisy and complex, contributing to more confusions for the person with Alzheimer's. Thus special care units provided a unique opportunity to personalize a simple environment to enhance the full potential of these residents. Usually admission criteria is based on ambulation, cognitive status, and the behavior and functional components of the resident who would most benefit from such an environment. Most provide a spacious, safe, locked environment for those individuals who wander and explore daily. In addition, cognitively stimulating programs and activities help maximize the resident's overall functional abilities.

The only true downfall of the Alzheimer's special care units is the frequent need to transfer patients from this assisted living-type facility, into the traditional nursing home as their condition deteriorates. Most licensing boards do not permit residents with additional medical needs to remain on a special care unit. However, allowing families to participate in the resident's plan of care is a vital link to a successful transfer.

Hospice Care Facilities

When a person is apparently in the final stages of illness, and death is imminent within six months, a Hospice Care Facility may be the most comforting answer to care. Hospice provides compassionate care for those who are near the end of a terminal illness like Alzheimer's disease.

Most hospices offer care by trained professionals both in the home setting, or in their care facility. Most hospice care is covered by Medicare.

Hospice staff is specifically trained to meet the special needs of end-stage dementia patients and their families. They take the time to understand the history of the disease and the caregivers' experiences from the onset. But most of all, they take the time to find ways to bring family members and patients together and establish quality time, on the patient's terms, for the final days.

It is true there are many care options from which to choose, but there are just as many consultants and counselors who are available to assist in those choices. It is imperative for primary caregivers to seek the help available to them and make informed choices regarding the placement and continuing care of a loved one who has Alzheimer's disease.

LISTEN TO MY HEART

Original Song by Nancy Lydic of Bonita Springs, Florida

One day when I was dreaming, I came up against a wall
The thing that I was thinking of was not a thought at all
You saw that I was fearful, so now catch me when I fall
Please understand my feelings and respond unto my call

CHORUS: Listen to my heart, instead of my head
Break it to me gently, the things that I've said
If I have to follow, I would rather be lead
So listen to my heart, instead of my head

I look deep into your eyes day after day
I know you love me but it's hard for you to say
I disappoint you in oh, so many ways
Please allow me to explain if I may

CHORUS

Now I am as far away as I could ever be
What is coming from my head isn't really even me
But still you care enough to show me love
And that's what sets me free
Thank You Heavenly Father from above
For helping us to see

CHORUS

Ending: Please listen to my heart, instead of my head.

(Shared with permission)

IN CONCLUSION

"LET THEM BE WHO THEY ARE NOW"

"I have to remind myself not to place my expectations and standards upon the person with Alzheimer's disease. I need to just let them be who they are now."

"The greatest need for a person with Alzheimer's is to know that someone is there for them—someone who will accept and love them just as they are now."

These insights from caregivers are pathfinders to understanding someone with Alzheimer's disease. This disease has the power to change lives, the lives of those who have it and of all who care for them.

It is said the much-loved illustrator Norman Rockwell was once asked if he considered himself a "realistic" painter. His answer was this, "Of course I am, but I paint 'reality' the way I'd like it to be."

Alzheimer's is, in reality, not the end of life as it was, but the beginning of life as it is. It is not the way we want it to be, but the way it is, for now. If all people will embrace this message, the burden of caregiving will be lightened for many What we have learned is Alzheimer's disease forever alters the brain, the memory, and the behavior. It is up to caregivers to change their approach, attitudes and modes of care to improve the lives of those afflicted with Alzheimer's disease. It is up to all of us to be compassionate, to "listen to their hearts."

We have heard the pleas of caregivers from around the world, from various walks of life. We are beginning to understand. There is so much more we need to learn, to share—about Alzheimer's disease.

RESOURCES

Organizations

The Alzheimer's Association / (ADRDA)
Alzheimer's Disease and Related Disorders Association
(800) 272-3900 or (312) 335-8700
919 North Michigan Avenue
Suite 1000
Chicago, IL 60611-1676
       The Alzheimer's Association was founded in 1980 and is the only national voluntary health organization dedicated both to research for the causes, treatments, cures and prevention of Alzheimer's disease, as well as to provide education and support for people with the disease, their families and caregivers. The Alzheimer's Association has a network of more than 200 chapters in 50 states working with over 35,000 volunteers providing programs and services to assist those with the disease and their families. A nationwide 24-hour information and referral line links families who need assistance with nearby Chapters.

Alzheimer's Disease Education and Referral Center
(800) 438-4380
P.O. Box 8250
Silver Springs, MD 20907-8250

Administration on Aging (AoA)
(800) 677-1116
330 Independence Avenue, SW
Washington, D.C. 20201

American Association of Homes and Services
for the Aging (AAHSA)
901 E Street NW
Suite 500
Washington, D.C. 20004-2037
An association of not-for-profit groups that provide health care, housing and community services to the elderly. It offers free brochures on choosing appropriate housing options for the elderly.

Area Agencies on Aging
Every state has an office on aging and most have networks of area agencies at the city, county, and/or multi-county level. Staff are prepared to help caregivers with any problems and make referrals to local resources. See your local phone directory for the number in your state.

Assisted Living Federation of America (ALFA)
(703) 691-8100
10300 Eaton Place
Suite 400
Fairfax, VA 22030
This organization represents over 4000 facilities and offers consumers guides on choosing an assisted living facility in your local area.

The Eldercare Locator
(800) 677-1116
A public service of the Administration on Aging, U.S. Department of Health and Human Services.

National Association for Home Care (NAHC)
228 Seventh Street, SE
Washington, D.C. 20003
This organization represents over 6000 agencies that offer home care services, hospice programs, and home care aid. They offer consumers' guides to home care.

The National Council on Aging, Inc. (NCOA)
(800) 375-1014
409 Third Street, SW
Second Floor
Washington, D.C. 20024

National Association for Music Therapy
301-589-3300

Literature

The 36-Hour Day: A Family Guide to Caring for Persons with Alzheimer's Disease, Related Dementing Illnesses, and Memory Loss in Later Life
By Nancy L. Mace and Peter V. Rabins
Johns Hopkins University Press, Baltimore, MD, 1991

Alzheimer's: A Caregiver's Guide and Source Book
By Howard Gruetzner
John Wiley & Sons, Inc.
New York, 1992

Alzheimer's Disease (37-page Report)
Harvard Medical School Health Publications Group
Boston, 1994

Flowers for Peggy
By Dr. Franklin K. Cassel
November, 1994

How To Care for Your Aging Parents, A Handbook for Adult Children
By Nora Jean Levin
Storm King Press, 1993.

How to Care for Your Aging Parents...and Still Have a Life of Your Own
By J. Michael Dolan,
Mulholland Pacific
Los Angeles, CA, 1992

Jill Came Tumbling After
One caregivers journey to acceptance
By Margo Piper
RitAmelia Press, 1995
Morriston, Florida

Living In the Labyrinth: A Personal Journey Through the Maze of Alzheimer's
By Diana Friel McGowin
Delacorte Press
New York, 1993

Long Distance Caregiving
By Angela Heath
American Source Books
Lakewood, CO, 1993

Seven Steps to Effective Parent Care
By Donna Cohen and Carl Eisdorfer
Putnam Books, New York, 1993

Articles

"A light side of Alzheimer's?" Conversation with Marc Silver and Deborah Hoffman, producer of documentary film "Complaints of a Dutiful Daughter." U.S. News & World Report, June 5, 1995

"Meeting the Spiritual Needs of the Cognitively Impaired"
Marty Richards. GENERATIONS Magazine, Fall, 1990

"Music Therapy with Caregivers and their Care Receivers in the Later Stages of Probable Alzheimer's Type Dementia." Alicia Ann Clair and Allison Grace Ebberts. Colmery-O'Neil Veterans Affairs Medical Center, Topeka, Kansas.

"Using AA principles and slogans as stress management tools for caregiver." R.P. Zahourek. Addictions Nursing Network, 1989 1(1):9-10.

Audio-Video Tapes

"Alzheimer's Disease at Time of Diagnosis"
Time/Life Medical
Narrated by C. Everett Koop, M.D.

"Complaints of a Dutiful Daughter"
Produced by Deborah Hoffman

The Internet

Amazon Book Store   http://www.amazon.com
Search: Alzheimer's Disease Book Titles

America's Guide Senior Infoserver   http://www.americasguide.com
A comprehensive index of living/service options for seniors.

Alzheimer's Association   http://www.alz.org

Alzheimers.com   http://alzheimers.com

The ALZHEIMER Page   http://www.biostat.wustl.edu

Caregiver Network   http://www.caregiver.on.ca

Pam Haisman, R.N., M.S.   http://www.pjh@chpublishers.com

�

ORDER FORM

Yes! Please send me _____ book(s):

"Alzheimer's Disease: Caregivers Speak Out"

NAME _____

ADDRESS _____

CITY_____ **STATE** _____ **ZIP** _____

I have enclosed:

$19.95 per book x _____ books	_____
Plus Shipping ($4.50 1 book; $3 ea. additional)	_____
SUBTOTAL	_____
Plus 6% sales tax for OH and FL residents	_____
TOTAL ENCLOSED	_____

PLEASE MAKE CHECKS PAYABLE TO: BookMasters, Inc.

SEND PAYMENT AND ORDER FORM TO:

> BookMasters, Inc.
> P.O. Box 388
> Ashland, OH 44805
> (419) 281-1802 Business Phone
> 1-800-247-6553 Book orders
> (419) 281-6883 FAX
> e-mail: order@bookmaster.com

Please allow 4 - 5 weeks for delivery.

For information on multiple book orders, special pricing, and/or seminar presentations, contact:

> Chippendale House Publishers
> P.O. Box 07155
> Fort Myers, FL 33919
> Fax: (941) 433-0421
> e-mail: pjh@chpublishers.com